A Revolution in Health Part 2: How to Take Charge of Your Health

John Neustadt, ND

Steve Pieczenik, MD, PhD

iUniverse, Inc.
New York   Bloomington

A Revolution in Health Part 2
How to Take Charge of Your Health

iUniverse books may be ordered through booksellers or by contacting:

iUniverse
1663 Liberty Drive
Bloomington, IN 47403
www.iuniverse.com
1-800-Authors (1-800-288-4677)

ISBN: 978-0-595-53216-2 (sc)
ISBN: 978-0-595-63277-0 (ebook)

Printed in the United States of America

iUniverse rev. date: 1/19/2009

Contents

What People Are Saying …

I am a fifty-nine-year-old male. I have been on a program for about four months now. I have to say that I do feel better overall. I contacted Dr. Neustadt because of ongoing quite uncomfortable joint pain and fatigue that would overcome me. I am a pretty strong guy, and work never bothered me, but the pain could knock me down.

I thought I knew what was causing it, and I had been taking different things to help. Nothing worked. Dr. Neustadt did an extensive blood workup and found so many things that I never have thought of. The problem that I thought was the cause was not even a factor. He pointed out all the things that were working against me, as well as the good things, and how it all works together. We also found that **I have a high concentration of heavy metals … lead and aluminum**. I was amazed. **The information that you find out is incredible.** We are currently working on the **fatigue**, for which I can say I am not having the bouts nearly as much anymore. He keeps an eye on your progress and monitors what you are taking and how you are feeling, and he adjusts it. I like that. I would highly recommend his program.

—Roger, Wisconsin

I just wanted to thank Dr. Neustadt for his excellent direction. I heard about him from a friend. I am fifty-nine-years old and was just not feeling good. I was **bloated, overweight, tired**; just thought that for my age, I should feel better. I believe I have taken every vitamin to "cure" this or that. And although I exercised, I had very little stamina. **I was tired of being tired out.**

I called Dr. Neustadt and he recommended the blood tests as the first step. I was just amazed at the results. They were not the routine tests that we have all been through—they gave indications of how my body was really behaving; such as what I was missing as far as amino acids, which I never thought about, because I thought I was eating right. They gave indications as to where you had too much of other things, even heavy metals. Dr. Neustadt put together a plan for me to follow. He sent me a packet that covered all the tests and what each indicator meant. We made an appointment to discuss the results. He went over every detail and why this works with this and why you feel like this. It was so thorough. **I went on the program (which was very easy to follow), and I can tell you that I feel great! The bloating is gone. I have dropped in size, and I have energy that I have never had. I love it.** The best part is really a total feeling of well-being. I just feel amazingly good! He also followed up with visits to discuss where I was and how I was feeling. I am very pleased. Thank you, Dr. Neustadt. And he has a great staff too.

—Dolores, Wisconsin

When I met Dr. Neustadt, I was immediately impressed by his knowledge and straightforward nature. Dr. Neustadt offers medical care that is founded in nature and supported by science. Having my BS in microbiology gives me direct knowledge of cellular function and chemistry. Therefore, in seeking naturopathic care, I was specifically looking for a practitioner who would couple natural health care and science in a way that would satisfy my scientific mind while healing me in a natural way. Dr. Neustadt fulfilled my needs, and his care exceeded my expectations.

My primary healthcare issue was **insomnia.** I had been struggling with this since I was eight years old. Dr. Neustadt performed a battery of blood and urine tests that identified deficiencies in my blood. The testing also determined what metabolites were not being properly used during the course of the metabolic process. The testing model that Dr. Neustadt uses is extraordinarily inclusive, and I would recommend it to anyone who is looking to get a solid baseline of his metabolic function (even if not ailing). That said, we were able to determine what was preventing me from sleeping. **We "rebooted" my system, which ultimately prompted my body to create what needs to be in the system to be balanced and healthy. I saw results almost immediately; this was the jumpstart my body needed.**

Dr. Neustadt also helped me after a fracture that ultimately required surgery. He prescribed a presurgical supplementation protocol that proved to be crucial in the healing process. The protocol dealt specifically with reducing the effects of the inflammatory process. I didn't realize that he would have something to help me in this way, but I'm glad I called; I'm fairly certain that my healing time was reduced because of the protocol.

Don't wait until you've exhausted all your options with traditional health care. Dr. Neustadt is wonderful at interfacing with your traditional healthcare practitioner. His goal is to find you relief, and your health is his first priority. If you are looking for someone who is bright, curious about you and your health history, and well rounded, Dr. Neustadt could be the fit you've been looking for.

—Diane, Montana

Three years ago, my then nine-year-old daughter suffered a severe **asthma attack** out of the blue, in the middle of a soccer match. From that day forward, asthma became a part of her life at school, at birthday parties, on camping trips … and everything changed for her. She gave up soccer, **gained weight**, became self-conscious, and seemed to have lost her previously strong immune system, catching every cold and flu, as well as struggling to get over them. First we fought it conventionally, and then we tried to get used to what seemed to be her new identity, with painful resignation.

What we both love and honor about Dr. John Neustadt is the way that he gave himself to the task of knowing us. Not only is he thorough and patient, he listens actively and interestedly, hears the implied but unspoken, and asks the questions that unravel the puzzle of each individual's health. He understands and trusts that his patients' knowledge about themselves is itself a powerful tool, a rare trait in any doctor. His faith in my daughter and me was the real beginning of our healing, and the rest followed. **My daughter is now asthma free**, and no one in our family doubts that the rest of her health is on its way back.

—Melissa, Montana

Over four years, I saw nine medical doctors, seeking help for my complicated condition. I have been suffering with severe gastroesophageal reflux (GERD). I had also been diagnosed with irritable bowel syndrome, for which there is no "known" cure (at least that is what conventional medical doctors will tell you). I would get severely and painfully bloated every time I ate, and I had diarrhea very frequently. I had a life-changing operation called a Nissen Fundoplication to help control my GERD symptoms. The operation pushed me deeper into a state of ill health. Over the last two years, the four MDs that I had been seeing continued to tell me that I was healthy, even though I had lost almost eighty pounds in that time. **The total cost of my medical care exceeded forty thousand dollars, and for all of this cost, I received basically no benefit.**

The MetaCT™ 400 test and MetaCT Program provided me with improvement in my condition, which I was told was not possible. For about a tenth of the cost of conventional treatments, Dr. Neustadt's treatments have reduced my IBS symptoms by over 90 percent. I no longer get bloated when I eat. I have not had diarrhea in almost two months. I no longer have hemorrhoids. On top of that, he helped me gain seventeen pounds in six weeks! I had been continually losing weight for two years. I am excited to see how much my health will continue to improve over the next few months.

I am so grateful that I found Dr. Neustadt. He has reminded me what life is like when you aren't in constant pain. He is an extremely intelligent, insightful, and caring man, and he is worth every dollar that you will spend on him as a healthcare provider.

—Steve, Washington

You can imagine my surprise when I received the reports from my lab study and discovered I was severely allergic to dairy products, egg yolks, egg whites, and peanuts. So, prior to my scheduled consultation, I immediately stopped consuming these items and foods that contained these ingredients.

Three days later, I felt like a new person. Most of the chronic muscle, bone, and joint aches I had been having for over ten years went away. I felt stronger, lighter on my feet, and, for the first time, I

tired out my children while playing with them outside. The "restless leg" condition I had been having at night stopped too. The slight depression I felt was lifted as well. I now sleep better, deeper, and wake up more refreshed. I have been to sleep studies and have seen many doctors, and nothing has helped as immediately and as noticeably as the removal of these foods from my diet.

—John, Alabama

In September 2006, I developed a condition that appeared to be a **seizure disorder**. After undergoing a series of tests, I was prescribed medications to make the seizures stop, but the side effects of those medications caused me to lose my memory, sometimes for several days at a time. Eventually, after even further testing, doctors concluded it was Pseudo Seizure Disorder. **I was told it was a psychological issue, and not at all neurological or medical in nature**.

Several months went by, and the symptoms worsened, to the point where I could barely walk, talk, or function at all. Then I was referred to **Dr. Neustadt, who was very dedicated and passionate about finding answers to my medical condition**. I went through extensive testing on a cellular level to see what was really going on in my body. After the testing, it was determined that I had an allergy to milk and was deficient in many of the essential vitamins and nutrients that I need. I was amazed that by day three of taking the nutritional supplements, my symptoms were gone. Since then, I have seen many other benefits to my health from making these changes. Dr. Neustadt worked with me to develop a weight loss program, which helped me lose thirty pounds. Now that my diet is better, my food cravings are mostly gone, and my mental and emotional states have also improved. **I strongly recommend anyone with medical issues to seek Dr. Neustadt's help** in uncovering what is going on at a cellular level. Thank you, Dr. Neustadt, for your compassion and help with getting me on a road to health.

—Darin, Montana

Introduction

This book is the second book in the Revolution in Health™ series. The first book, *A Revolution in Health through Nutritional Biochemistry*, was written by the authors in 2007. They now follow up that work with this groundbreaking book, *A Revolution in Health Part 2: How to Take Charge of Your Health*. In these books, they describe how they have put into practice more than one hundred years of research, and how you can use this information to revolutionize your life.

How often have you heard the words, "There's nothing more we can do. Take this pill and come back and see us?" How many of you have felt angry, disappointed, depressed, and confused—feeling simply lost while your suffering from an ailment continues unabated? You can no longer trust the medical system. The doctor you trusted for a long time seems lost too. And the pills either do nothing, or may be helpful but have definite side effects.

So you start searching the internet or looking through reference books, and you're overwhelmed by conflicting opinions and studies you cannot truly understand or trust. You call your friends or neighbors and ask what they would do if they were in a similar situation. Even then, the answers are not compelling. You then turn to anything that seems to be an alternative solution, and you may start doing energy medicine, kinesiology, spiritual counseling, or other things you think may help. It's understandable that you try new ways, and because you pay a lot of money and want to prove to your skeptical family or friends that the solution you found works, you try to convince yourself that it does as well. But unfortunately, you know within yourself that it's not working, and you feel more angry, frustrated, and depressed. What happens is that you feel either immobilized or overwhelmed, and that this is "just the way it is," and you resign yourself to suffering.

This is exactly what happened with Dr. Pieczenik (pronounced P-chen-ik). For years, he experienced shortness of breath. His physician didn't consider it important and thought he might just be allergic to his daughter's cat. In the latter part of December 2007, Dr. Pieczenik went to see his physician on the East Coast, who was an extremely competent and accessible internist. Dr. Pieczenik went to this doctor complaining of walking pneumonia. What this means is that he was experiencing a dry, hacking cough. He had never suffered from allergies or mature onset asthma, so he knew these weren't the cause of his problem. He was not suffering from fevers, body aches, or any other symptoms. All Dr. Pieczenik wanted was to see his physician so that she could place a stethoscope on his chest and determine whether she heard any unusual noises that might signify that he had pneumonia. While all doctors are trained to do this, and he could have done this for himself, he wanted to get an objective evaluation from his own physician. Walking pneumonia, if he did have it, is a simple diagnosis with a simple solution—prescribe antibiotics.

Instead of receiving the service Dr. Pieczenik expected, which should have only been a quick ten- to fifteen-minute visit, he spent over an hour and a half in the doctor's office, taking laboratory tests that were totally unnecessary, with the exception of a blood test for the organism *Mycoplasma pneumoniae*, which is diagnostic for walking pneumonia, and which Dr. Pieczenik had to ask for himself. In addition to all this, he never once actually saw a physician, despite his insistence that one come in the room to evaluate him. The consistent response from laboratory technicians and secretaries to Dr. Pieczenik's requests to see a doctor, which, by the way, he thought he was going to be doing when he made his "doctor's appointment," was to wait for the tests. He never did actually even speak to a physician, nor did any doctor perform a physical examination and listen to his lungs. He requested that the results from the *Mycoplasma* blood test be faxed to him immediately after completion of the test so that he might have a diagnosis. Out of simple frustration and fear, Dr. Pieczenik did not wait to receive his test results, which he didn't even receive for three weeks, and even then, no physician called or inquired as to his health. The test, by the way, was positive. Out of simple frustration and fear, Dr. Pieczenik did not wait to receive his test results (which he didn't even receive for three weeks, and even then, no physician called or inquired as to his health. The test, by the way, was positive) to treat himself with antibiotics. For all this, he received a bill for nearly one thousand dollars.Dr. Pieczenik returned to Bozeman, Montana, and told his partner, Dr. Neustadt, of his experience.

Interestingly enough, at the same time Dr. Pieczenik was having his problems with the medical system on the East Coast, Dr. Neustadt was having his own difficulties. Dr. Neustadt's wife needed her annual pelvic examination and blood work. The pelvic examination is commonly called a PAP smear, which diagnosis the risk for cervical cancer in women. Every medical society and medical school mandates that this pelvic examination be required for every sexually active woman. When Dr. Neustadt's wife went to her board-certified OB/GYN physician, she supplied the receptionist with her insurance card. For his wife, his young son, and himself, Dr. Neustadt paid $350 per month for health insurance with a five-thousand-dollar deductible. Like many families, Dr. Neustadt rightfully assumed that this policy covered routine examinations. And that even if they weren't covered procedures done by licensed physicians, they would at least count toward their deductible. He and his wife were shocked to discover that her doctor's appointment and the tests were not covered—$156 for the gynecologist visit, plus $51 for the PAP smear test to be processed. They were even more distressed to learn that this out-of-pocket expense would not count toward their deductible!

Drs. Neustadt and Pieczenik concluded that the healthcare system is in no way oriented toward prevention or even treatment of mild, routine conditions. Instead, it's a disease-based healthcare system that is dysfunctional and only capable of properly treating medical disasters such as heart attacks, car accidents, and cancer. In short, the entire medical system is geared toward acute trauma and disasters, not routine medical care or prevention of disease. It is not an accident that most physicians end up in specialty care, such as hand surgeons, medical oncologists and plastic surgeons, because that's where the insurance reimbursements or high-cost cash procedures are. Family physicians are decreasing in numbers as their incomes are decreasing due to liability insurance and health insurance companies continually decreasing the amount of reimbursement.

Drs. Neustadt and Pieczenik began asking friends and patients throughout the country about their experiences with doctors and health insurance companies. More than 90 percent of the fifty or so people with whom they spoke related similar experiences: inaccessible and overworked physicians; expensive tests that seemed unnecessary in many cases, had the doctor simply taken the time to see the patient and conduct even a cursory interview and physical examination; and frustrations with a bureaucracy that shuttles people to different specialists and locations without actually providing answers or benefit.

These people experienced exactly what Dr. Pieczenik did: complete frustration, disgust, and mistrust.

Our healthcare system is melting down. It's broken, and there is no way to improve it from the inside. Instead, Drs. Pieczenik and Neustadt realized that the only solution would come from the consumers themselves. People must be educated to understand how they can take charge of their own health care to be their own best advocate, reduce their frustration and healthcare costs, and improve their health. That is the essence of this book. Together, Drs. Neustadt and Pieczenik decided to formulate a plan that any individual can use to manage his own health care, since few doctors or insurance companies will ever fully be there for the patient.

This book is a map to help you navigate yourself to better health. By completing simple steps and learning the basics of your own biology and healthcare needs, you take control of your own health care.

First, readers need to learn basic principles of your body and how it works. Second, the authors want readers to understand how those elements interrelate structurally and functionally to determine their health. Third, you will learn about basic medical tests that you need. Fourth, the authors give readers the unique opportunity to order their own tests. Fifth, Drs. Neustadt and Pieczenik provide a twelve-step program to empower you to improve and promote your health through diet, lifestyle, and proper medical testing. Why twelve steps? Because the authors know from previous experience and addiction programs that twelve steps is the most effective way to achieve lasting results.

The authors dedicate this book to everyone who has felt the way they have felt—trapped in a healthcare system that is not dedicated to helping people, but rather to making money for insurance companies. They view you, the reader, as a consumer of information and knowledge, who is seeking the necessary tools and ingredients to improve your own health.

Health is a journey of self-discovery. The authors feel honored to be part of the reader's journey, and hope that readers will let Drs. Neustadt and Pieczenik know about their experiences, as well as what information they might provide in future books to best help you and your family.

Chapter 1:
Understanding Health and Disease

Health is a sense of well-being that is defined by three different time elements. The past defines what your family and you have had, and may provide information about your risk for future illnesses. For example, one of the most important predictors of breast cancer in women is if the woman's mother had breast cancer. Similarly, if a parent or a sibling had or has any cancers, diabetes, or heart disease, you are automatically in a higher risk category than people whose immediate family does not have these conditions. It may be that you have a genetic predisposition to these conditions, but more likely it's because family members tend to follow the same lifestyle and dietary pattern—lack of exercise, poor diets, and high stress. Research suggests that 80 percent of large bowel, breast, and prostate cancers are caused by poor nutrition, physical inactivity, and obesity.[1, 2] And the predominant causes of heart disease and diabetes are the same.

When we hear people exhibit a fatalistic attitude by saying that their heart disease or any other condition is just "genetic," most of the time it's simply a rationale for them to not take responsibility for their own health. The reality is different. While genetics are important, lifestyle and dietary factors become even more important as we age. Rationalization is an underappreciated dynamic that is far more powerful than people realize. Rationalizations allow people to explain away their responsibilities for taking care of their own health. For this reason, we felt even more compelled to write this book. If nothing else, we are trying to break through people's rationalizations and inertia to help motivate and empower them to identify and break bad habits and excuses.

Your own past medical history provides extremely important information about what your current condition may be, but it also indicates what you may be at risk of getting in the future. For example, if you frequently suffered from ear infections as a child, and were put on repeated courses of antibiotics, you may now be at increased risk for intestinal infections called intestinal dysbiosis. Bacteria commonly cause these infections, and when caused by yeast, they're referred to as intestinal candidiasis. Symptoms of this condition include gas and bloating; postnasal drip; headaches; brain fog (difficulty processing information); diarrhea or constipation; and in more severe cases, rashes, muscle, and joint aches.

Similarly, if you have had a history of any cancer, you are at an extremely elevated risk of another cancer. But if you follow a whole-foods, plant-based diet that is low in fat; exercise; and practice stress reduction, you may reduce your risk of another cancer. There are also tests, which we will discuss in the latter part of this book, that you should take at specific intervals to monitor yourself and stack the deck in your favor.

The final crucial components of evaluating your health risks have to do with understanding and taking inventory of your environmental exposures, dietary and lifestyle considerations, and medications. Environmental contamination has become a serious public health problem. Eighteen drinking water studies have linked aluminum level to elevated risks of Alzheimer's disease and cognitive impairment in the elderly.[3] Arsenic exposure is a risk factor for prostate cancer, cadmium for bladder cancer, and parabens for breast cancer. Between fifty thousand and one hundred thousand synthetic chemicals are being produced commercially around the world.[4]

Well-functioning biochemistry, which promotes health, vitality and the general sense of well-being, can be altered by stress, exercise, pharmaceuticals, nutritional deficiencies, and toxic exposures to heavy metals and solvents. Exposure to these determinants of biochemical health, which cause symptoms such as headaches, strokes, depression, fatigue, cancer, eczema, and fibromyalgia can be tested for and corrected. This is done using sophisticated biochemical tests that provide the data for creating customized programs that promote health by optimizing diet and lifestyle, removing environmental contaminants and providing the underlying nutrients for the body to function optimally.

How Do You Know Your Present Condition?

Understanding your present state of health is as much a subjective feeling as it is an objective analysis. The first question you need to ask yourself is simply, "How do I feel?" It's as basic as that. And yet this question is extremely penetrating. When people ask themselves exactly how they feel, they tend to rationalize away anything negative about their physical or mental health. Recognizing that they don't feel well can be uncomfortable for people because it places them in a vulnerable position. Most people, including your doctors, do not like to feel vulnerable, and so they compensate by rationalizing that there's nothing else to do.

On a more personal level, in the winter months of early 2005 Dr. Pieczenik suffered from a chronic dry, hacking, quite annoying cough that had been going on for months. Not knowing why he had it, he simply dismissed it as a side effect of the dry, cold Montana air—or figured that it was possibly caused by his daughter's cat. In order to ameliorate his cough, he purchased humidifiers for his home, avoided the cat as much as possible, and had all his carpets and drapes professionally cleaned. He also had the cat shaved. He was hopeful that this would give him the relief he sought. However, much to his own amazement, his cough got worse, not better.

Dr. Pieczenik knew very well from the outset that a persistent dry cough like his could be an important warning sign for walking pneumonia, mature onset asthma, pulmonary hypertension, or congestive heart failure. He was in his early sixties when the cough began, and he knew clinically that he should be worked up to rule out the worst-case scenario. However, his denial of the more serious implications of his symptoms is simply a common psychological dynamic that all people use in dealing with their health.

When he literally could not ski on the novice runs anymore at our local ski resort, Bridger Bowl, because he was so short of breath, he flew to the east coast where he was evaluated by top specialists in Pulmonology and Cardiology. This included a chest X-ray, cardiac stress test, and pulmonary function tests. He and the other doctors were shocked to discover that Dr. Pieczenik had a 25 percent oxygen deficit, which meant that he really should not have been alive. Fortunately, he did not have congestive heart failure, walking pneumonia, or pulmonary hypertension. What he did have was mature onset asthma, for which his colleagues offered prescription steroids and a bronchodilator inhaler.

Since steroids and inhalers have been the most common therapy for these symptoms for many years, Dr. Pieczenik asked his doctors, "How come the treatment of exertion asthma has not changed in forty years?" Dr. Pieczenik did not accept the answers he was given. He felt that neither doctor understood the underlying causes of the problem. His diagnosis was relegated to the wastebasket of medicine—the chronic we-don't-really-understand-why catchall diagnosis. So, in turn, the catchall treatment was to prescribe steroids, which are handed out as though they are candy. Nevertheless, Dr. Pieczenik tried the steroids and inhaler and found them totally ineffectual, as he had expected. In fact, when he took the steroids, they kept him awake for more than seventy-two hours, a documented side effect of these drugs. Unfortunately, his physicians had neglected to tell him of this side effect.

By chance, Dr. Pieczenik had met Dr. Neustadt, a naturopathic physician with a specialization in nutritional biochemistry, a couple of years earlier at Sweet Pea Festival, an annual summer arts and food festival in Bozeman. At that time, Dr. Pieczenik mentioned to Dr. Neustadt that he had a breathing difficulty that had not existed earlier in his life, and Dr. Neustadt casually said that Dr. Pieczenik probably had a decrease in epinephrine production. Epinephrine is a chemical in the body that, among other things, helps to dilate the lungs so people can breathe. Still skeptical of Dr. Neustadt's explanation, Dr. Pieczenik continued to endure his condition. But one day he made an appointment with Dr. Neustadt and agreed to a comprehensive biochemical evaluation.

His workup included a standard medical evaluation with a physical examination, but Dr. Neustadt also ordered a series of blood and urine tests to analyze more than four hundred variables of biochemical function. These tests revealed that the underlying cause of Dr. Pieczenik's problem was low copper, which prevented the production of epinephrine, a bronchodilator hormone in the body. And that's how Dr. Pieczenik became interested in educating people about how they can take their personal health care into their own hands.

Dr. Neustadt's interest in taking charge of his own health also grew out of personal frustration with the medical system. He was working in high tech in Seattle for various companies, such as Boeing, Microsoft, and assorted start-up software companies, when he began to get sick, feeling depressed and fatigued. His first impulse was to deny this situation and throw himself ever further into work. Dr. Neustadt did what most people do: he avoided dealing with his problems and masked them by being even more outgoing, trying to work more intensely, and climbing the corporate ladder. And he was also a "weekend warrior," doing extreme sports such as rock climbing and mountain climbing. Even then, he realized that the symptoms would not simply disappear.

Dr. Neustadt finally went to see his physician, a kind, general practitioner. The doctor spoke with Dr. Neustadt for a few minutes, ran a simple blood test to evaluate Dr. Neustadt's thyroid gland, and told him probably nothing was wrong. When Dr. Neustadt tried to ask additional questions, the physician got annoyed. When the lab test returned, the doctor said it was negative. Still frustrated, Dr. Neustadt knew something was wrong. He had heard of Bastyr University, a naturopathic medical school in Seattle, Washington. He made an appointment at the teaching clinic and was fortunate to have the chief medical officer, Dr. Jamey Wallace, ND, supervising the medical students for that shift. Dr. Wallace and the students spent an hour with Dr. Neustadt, discussing his symptoms, lifestyle, profession, and hobbies. They really took the time to get to know him. At the end of the intake, Dr. Wallace turned to Dr. Neustadt and said, "The goal of naturopathic medicine is to treat the underlying cause, and I think the major cause of your complaints is your work. I think you need to quit your job."

Dr. Neustadt had discussed with Dr. Wallace and the student clinicians his interests in medicine and his background in botany and biochemistry. Like many people, Dr. Neustadt was subconsciously just looking to confirm and approve what he already knew. The next week, Dr. Neustadt quit his job and began applying to medical school.

The rest is history. Dr Neustadt went on to become one of the top students at Bastyr University, and soon after, he opened a successful practice in Bozeman, Montana.

When Dr. Neustadt opened his clinic, Montana Integrative Medicine (MIM), he decided that he would provide the same medical care and experience for his patients that he would want to have if he were a patient. He continued his research into the underlying biochemical causes of disease and began running tests on patients to help them. Soon after starting the clinic, he joined Dr. Pieczenik in creating their nutraceutical company, Nutritional Biochemistry, Inc. (NBI, www.nbihealth.com), and their testing and consulting company, NBI Testing and Consulting Corp. (NBITC, www.nbitesting.com). Their philosophy was to afford the patient the greatest opportunity to learn about himself through testing, and then to promote the patient's health by correcting the underlying biochemical and nutritional causes of symptoms and diseases. The simplest way to do this was to provide pharmaceutical-grade dietary supplements with the dose and form of nutrients shown in clinical trials and basic research to work. When Dr. Neustadt was unable to find an existing formulation that could help his patients, Drs. Neustadt and Pieczenik would create it themselves.

In doing this work over several years, Drs. Picczenik and Neustadt realized that there was a real need to educate the public directly about how they can take charge of their own health. And that people need to understand the basic testing that they can request to help themselves. Many people are struggling with no health insurance, high deductibles, and difficulty getting an appointment with a doctor who will spend the time with them that they deserve.

The Polypharmacy Phenomenon

Polypharmacy means taking multiple drugs at the same time. Usually people end up taking five or more different medications for the major chronic, degenerative diseases, such as high cholesterol, diabetes, high blood pressure, depression, and arthritis. They may be taking Lipitor, Lisinopril, Lexapro, Metformin, Celebrex, and others. What each of these drugs does is to attempt to treat a symptom. Not one of these drugs actually treats the underlying causes of these symptoms, and it doesn't stop or reverse the underlying condition, which progressively worsens with aging.

What is happening is that doctors are not looking at you as a whole entity. Instead, they are chopping you up into piecemeal components and treating each component separately, as if they are not connected. The analogy is that if you are hemorrhaging, the doctor is putting small bandages on you instead of identifying and correcting the underlying cause of bleeding. Now, admittedly, the medical field has done an excellent job with dealing with acute crises or traumas. Conventional medicine has had a much harder time being able to understand the degenerative aging process, as well as how it pertains to the entire body specifically. Conventionally trained physicians are not taught to integrate different body systems and to think or treat people holistically. Nor do they receive education concerning nutrition or lifestyle factors in disease and aging. They are experts in drugs and surgery, but even then, the majority of the time, these interventions merely treat symptoms, not the underlying causes.

There's an alternative way to approach your health. The first step in doing this is to understand which tests you may need and how to get them. In effect, you need to become your best-informed advocate because we are all now dealing with a healthcare system that is rife with arrogance, ignorance, and incompetence.

But don't despair. Like us, you have to find the way your own way and enter the new world of managing your own health care. Admittedly, it sounds like an awesome and overwhelming task. But we will help you through baby steps to navigate this system so that you become extremely comfortable with your body, knowledge, and most importantly, with how to treat your body accordingly.

How Medicine Defines You

Conventional medicine has created a system of diagnosis that meets its needs and the needs of the pharmaceutical and insurance industries. The reductionist model used by physicians is based largely on symptoms, rarely on causality. For example, a diagnosis of depression is merely based on symptoms (e.g., you tell the doctor your energy is low, you feel hopeless or helpless, etc.) and signs, which are what the physician observes (e.g., flat affect, slow speech, etc.). There can be many causes of depression. Doctors will usually only do a cursory evaluation, which might include a thyroid test and a complete blood count and a serum chemistries, and ask you if you're not sleeping well, if you're under excessive stress, or if there are some life situations causing your depression.

If those tests and questions don't confirm any particular diagnosis other than depression, then doctors frequently just prescribe an antidepressant. Many times the antidepressant really doesn't help, and in fact may compound the depression even more so. A January 17, 2008, report from the *New England Journal of Medicine* (NEJM) titled "Selective Publication of Antidepressant Trials and Its Influence on Apparent Efficacy" revealed that antidepressant medications only work 40 to 50 percent of the time. Manufacturers of all antidepressant medications currently on the market biased their study data and did not publish data that went against their corporate interests. The effectiveness of these medications was thus artificially inflated by nearly 70 percent in the case of Serzone, and by 64 percent in the case of Zoloft. Consequently, doctors and patients are getting a distorted view of the usefulness of antidepressants like Effexor, Zoloft, Welbutrin, Paxil, Remeron, and Prozac.

Many of the underlying causes of depression, however, can be tested for and quickly corrected. The biochemical pathways in the body that influence mood—and how toxins, infections, and allergies affect mood—are all well defined. What, then, are the common underlying causes of depression? The questions physicians ask and the tests they run are important to order to rule out low thyroid function and emotional and lifestyle factors. However, this line of reasoning captures less than 1 percent of the important underlying causes of depression. These causes include deficiencies in amino acids, magnesium, manganese, iron, B-complex vitamins, coenzyme Q10, and alpha lipoic acid; accumulation of toxic metals such as lead or mercury; problems regulating blood sugar regulation due to any of these nutritional deficiencies and poor diet; food allergies; and infections, commonly intestinal infections.

Nutrients that feed these pathways, not drugs, are what are required to improve mood. Therefore, there's no incentive for the pharmaceutical industry to develop effective treatments because it goes against their financial interests. And since the pharmaceutical industry defines most of the medical education in this country, conventionally educated physicians never study the underlying biochemical causes of diseases.

While the effects of specific nutrients and pathways of depression are well documented (see figures 1.1a and 1.1b), conventional medicine ignores them. Instead of providing customized treatments based on a person's specific biochemical needs, conventional medicine adopts a one-size-fits-all approach to depression by prescribing antidepressant medications. These medications fall into two classes—selective serotonin reuptake inhibitors (SSRIs) and selective serotonin and norepinephrine reuptake inhibitors (SNRIs). Examples of SSRI medications include Zoloft, Lexapro, Celexa, and Prozac, and an example of a SNRI medication is Welbutrin.

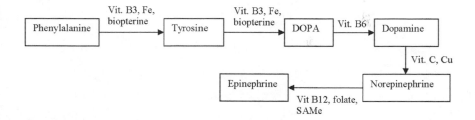

Figure 1.1a. Low dopamine and epinephrine can cause fatigue and depression. The SNRI medications work on this pathway to artificially increase dopamine and epinephrine, but people can be deficient in phenylalanine, tyrosine, or vitamins and minerals required for dopamine and epinephrine production. When testing reveals the exact deficiency, nutrients can be supplied to aid the body in producing its own dopamine and serotonin naturally, without medications. Moreover, the natural approach is nearly devoid of any risk for side effects, while the SNRI medications carry significant risk of serious side effects. Abbreviations: Vit. B3 = Vitamin B3; Fe = iron; Vit. B6 = Vitamin B6; Vit. C = Vitamin C; Cu = Copper; SAMe = S-adenosylmethionine.

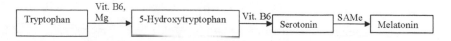

Figure 1.1b. The essential amino acid L-tryptophan and vitamin B6 are required for the production of serotonin and melatonin. Serotonin helps control mood, and melatonin helps people sleep. The SSRI and SNRI medications increase serotonin by decreasing its breakdown

instead of providing the raw materials for effective serotonin production. Abbreviations: Mg = Magnesium; SAMe = S-adenosyl methionine; Vit. B6 = Vitamin B6.

Many people turn to stimulants and short-term solutions to lift their spirits and energy, such as alcohol, sugar, caffeine, cocaine, methamphetamines, and Ritalin. These substances provide brief relief from the symptoms of fatigue, but in effect, they make the underlying causes of the problems worse. For example, sugar directly stimulates a release of serotonin in the central nervous system, thereby lifting mood, and it also provides fuel for energy production. The problem is that eating sugar also stimulates insulin release because insulin's job is to help move sugar from the bloodstream and into cells that use the sugar for energy. But when this happens, blood sugar drops and the person becomes hypoglycemic (having low blood sugar), which manifests itself in the symptoms of irritability, restlessness, insomnia, fatigue, and depression.[5] The paradox here is that even though people feel fatigued, they also feel restless and may have insomnia because of the subsequent low serotonin and melatonin.

There is another irony here. Most people who feel depressed and tired often drink alcohol to sleep, but within a few hours, they wake up with increased irritability, restlessness, and insomnia, which can become intractable since the more they feel these symptoms the more they want to drink in order to eliminate them. The alcohol itself is a central nervous system depressant, but it's also just fermented sugar, and alcoholic beverages therefore contain high amounts of carbohydrates. The rebound effect on mood and energy is explained by the same mechanisms as sugar itself. When blood sugar drops too low during sleep, it stimulates the release of cortisol and epinephrine. These hormones cause the release of stored sugars in the body to raise blood sugar, but they also wake a person up. The more someone drinks and the more someone eats sugar to lift his mood, the more his problems are compounded because of the resultant hypoglycemia.

An additional factor is that as people eat more sugar and drink more alcohol, the consumption of nutrient-dense foods containing essential vitamins, minerals, and amino acids decreases. So if the cause for depression and fatigue is a deficiency in the compounds required for healthy neurotransmitter production, masking the symptoms by consuming sugar, alcohol, and other substances that provide a short-term boost in mood and energy actually worsens the depression and fatigue. This becomes a vicious cycle that people have great difficulty breaking out of because the withdrawal effects can be more severe than the addiction.

The diagnosis of depression, just like other diagnoses such as irritable bowel syndrome, arthritis, asthma, obesity, and restless leg syndrome is simply based on gross signs and symptoms. The analogy the authors like to use is that if you're in an airplane flying over a large city, you may be able to tell that there's a traffic jam on the highway, but the reason for it remains a mystery. Similarly, your symptoms are the fifty-thousand-foot view, but biochemical evaluations can likely answer the crucial question, "Doctor, but *why* do I feel this way?" Unfortunately, most patients are so relieved once they receive a diagnosis that they usually don't go beyond that point and ask, "Why? What are the underlying causes, and what can be done about them?" And doctors seldom ever go beyond their diagnoses to ask themselves why.

Chapter 2:
Taking Your Health Inventory

Most of you are probably not physicians, and that's okay. Nor are you going to be physicians after reading this book once or twice. You do not need to memorize or absorb all the information in this book. Instead, it can serve as a map for you to navigate through your problems and your body in a way that has a logical sequence and is accessible to you as a reader.

What do we mean by logical? The authors discussed different ways to organize this book. One of the ways we looked at presenting this is through a systematic analysis of signs and symptoms of different organ systems. For example, the brain has many different anatomic parts, each one exhibiting its own signs and symptoms. And likewise with the eyes, ears, throat, stomach, and other organs. Trust us when we tell you that this would have been a textbook of about sixteen hundred pages, akin to what a medical student must study and learn.

So we decided to discuss the most common symptoms that most physicians see in specific age groups. We've also listed routine tests that a physician would order for specific age groups. People fall into two major categories. One is those people whose health is generally good and they want to maintain that. Unfortunately, this is the minority of people. The authors have found that, instead, most people are reactive and not proactive. That is, they don't tend to pay attention to their health until they begin to have problems. Once you have symptoms, then the approach to your health is quite different. Part of taking charge of your own health is becoming more proactive, if you already are not that way. Many diseases can be effectively treated, and even reversed, using natural, nontoxic means such as changes in diet, lifestyle, and dietary supplements. However, any good physician will tell you that the first thing to do before starting treatment is to get a good diagnosis. From the diagnosis flows all the possible treatment options.

Healthy Individuals with No Major Risk Factors

If you feel well and do not have any complaints, such as depression, fatigue, irritable bowel syndrome, or major risk factors for disease, start with this first section. Major risk factors for disease include being overweight; having a sedentary lifestyle (not exercising); having grandparents, mother, father, sister, or brother with a history of cancers, diabetes, heart disease, or other medical conditions.

This section defines which tests are commonly recommended at specific intervals for specific age groups and genders in people with no major risk factors for disease. These routine tests are what any physician would likely order for a routine checkup. The one caveat here is that this testing schedule is for people with no known risk factors for diseases, which, unfortunately, include the minority of people (table 2.1).

Table 2.1. Routine physical Exams and Tests for Low-Risk Patients.

Age	Physical Exams and Tests
18-39	• **Women and Men:** ✓ Monthly: skin check (moles and birthmarks) ✓ Annually: Dental exam and cleaning, blood pressure (can be done at most local drug stores for free), skin check (moles and birthmarks) ✓ Twice during your twenties: cholesterol • **Women:** monthly self breast exam, yearly pelvic exam and pap smear • **Men:** monthly self testicular exam
40-65	• **Women and Men:** ✓ Monthly: skin check (moles and birthmarks) ✓ Annually: dental exam and cleaning every year, blood pressure (can be done for free at most drug stores), cholesterol (if you have a previous abnormal test), rectal exam and stool guiac test for colorectal cancer screening ✓ Every one to five years: physical exam ✓ Every two years: eye exam after age of 40, including a check for glaucoma. ✓ Every three years: fasting blood glucose to screen for diabetes ✓ Every three to five years: flexible sigmoidoscopy beginning at age 50 ✓ Every five years: cholesterol (if elevated, check yearly) ✓ At 40 years old: lean body mass measurement, then every 5 years; nutritional evaluation by a nutritionist • **Women:** monthly self breast exam; yearly pelvic exam and pap smear; mammogram every 1 to 2 years once over the age of 40 and yearly after age of 50; baseline bone density scan at age 60 • **Men:** yearly rectal exam after age of 50; yearly PSA blood test for prostate cancer risk after 50; baseline bone density scan at age 60
Over the age of 65	• **Women and Men:** ✓ Monthly: Skin check (moles and birthmarks) monthly self exams ✓ Annually: Dental exam and cleaning, hearing test, blood pressure (can be done for free at most drug stores), physical exam, rectal exam and stool guiac test to screen for colorectal cancer ✓ Every two years: eye exam, including check for glaucoma ✓ Every three years: fasting blood glucose to screen for diabetes ✓ Every three to five years: cholesterol (if normal, more frequently if abnormal), flexible sigmoidoscopy to screen for polyps and colorectal cancer (or colonoscopy every 10 years) • **Women:** monthly self breast exam, pelvic exam and pap smear every 1 to 3 years; mammogram yearly • **Men:** yearly rectal exam and PSA test to screen for prostrate cancer

*If moles or birthmarks are changing in color or size, see a Dermatologist.

Healthy Individuals with Risk Factors: The 80/20 Rule

Although you may be feeling well, you may still be at increased risk for diseases based on your family history, your lifestyle, and your own personal history. For example, if your mother, father, sister, or brother has a history of colorectal cancer, diabetes, obesity, or cardiovascular disease, you are automatically at increased risk for these conditions. If you are a woman whose mother had breast cancer, you are automatically in a higher risk category for getting breast cancer than a woman whose mother never had breast cancer. But you can change that risk.

The authors have often heard from patients, "My father, brother, and uncles all have heart disease and died at a young age, so it's genetic." This fatalistic attitude is essentially the way many people rationalize not having to take care of themselves, or learn how to take care of themselves. Even if you have a genetic predisposition to a disease, the irony is that genetics does not mean you will absolutely get a disease.

Except for extreme cases, genetics *only predisposes you to a disease*. Genes create proteins in your body used for all biological processes. When someone is genetically predisposed, it means that the proteins they create may not function adequately. However, genes are constantly being turned on and off, and are no longer even considered the major determinants of health. There are thirty to forty thousand different protein-coding genes in humans,[6] but there are more than five hundred thousand different proteins in the human body.[7]

Surprisingly, more important than genetics for determining disease are dietary, lifestyle, and environmental factors. Each of these variables changes your biochemistry and can push you in a direction of health or disease. This concept is so important that the authors want to illustrate it to you in a concrete way.

Whatever you do in your day-to-day life alters your biochemistry and your physiology (how your body functions). Biochemistry mediates what happens between the outside and inside worlds. What the authors would like to do is to help you change your biochemistry in such a way that it moves you in the direction of health and not disease.

Like patients, frequently when doctors say, "It's genetic," the comment is often a rationalization by physicians to exempt themselves from the responsibility of not pushing the boundaries of their own knowledge. Physicians do not have the time, curiosity, or training to research the underlying mechanisms of diseases. The authors cannot really blame them.

The real culprit is what the authors consider the evil axis of the pharmaco-insurance-medical school industry. This alliance overall does more harm than good. This pressure on physicians to see more patients in less time and prescribe more medications is immense. Physicians now see about forty patients every day. That's nearly twelve minutes per patient. On average, within eighteen seconds, a physician will interrupt a patient describing his symptoms. In that short time, many doctors decide on the likely diagnosis and best treatment.

Do you really think any physician has the time and energy necessary to understand the underlying causes of your symptoms and disease? There's no financial incentive for physicians to go beyond those twelve minutes. Secondly, and more importantly, physicians are overworked and can physically only handle so much.

So when a doctor says to a woman, "Your mother had breast cancer, and therefore you will likely have it; it's genetic," he is usually speaking from the point of a view of incomplete knowledge and an inaccurate medical model that scares women without educating or empowering them. While genetic predisposition for the development of breast cancer is important, it plays less of a role than most people realize. Genetic factors alone explain only approximately 5 percent of all cancers. The BRCA1 (breast cancer gene 1) genes have been linked to the development of breast cancer, but this genetic mutation explains only about 5 percent of breast cancer cases in women younger than forty years old, 2 percent of cases in women aged forty to forty-nine years, and 1 percent of cases in women aged fifty to seventy years.[8] Much more important for decreasing a woman's risk for breast cancer risk are eating a low-fat diet, exercising regularly, and testing for the ratios of different estrogens in the body.

Liver detoxification pathways exert major influences over the risk for and development of cancers. One such pathway metabolizes estrogen. Estrogen can be metabolized predominantly via two pathways that produce 2-hydroxyestrogen (2-OHE) and 16-hydroxyestrogen (16-OHE). The former protects against the development of breast and uterine cancers, while 16-OHE increases the risk. Epidemiological studies show that a low 2-to-16 hydroxyestrogen ratio (low amounts of 2-OHE and higher amounts of 16-OHE) increases a woman's risk of breast cancer by 45 percent.[9] This ratio can be determined by a simple urine test, and it is a much more powerful indicator of breast cancer risk than the BRCA1 genotype because the ratio of estrogens is a *functional* indicator of what is actually happening in the body while the genotype is not functional.

The enzymes that metabolize 16-OHE are *constitutive*, meaning that they are static and cannot be modified. Therefore, if a woman's 16-OHE level is elevated, this cannot be changed. But it's the ratio of

2-OHE to 16-OHE that's important, not the absolute concentration of each individual metabolite. The 2-OHE pathway is *inducible*; its activity can be increased so that 2-OHE production can be increased. This can be accomplished by consuming higher amounts of cruciferous vegetables, such as broccoli and cauliflower, and also by taking a dietary supplement containing adequate amounts of diindolylmethane (DIM).[10] Altering this ratio may decrease a woman's risk of developing breast and uterine cancer.

Without trying to overwhelm you, the bottom line is that taking charge of your health is the best way to help yourself. No doctor or pill will do as much for you as you can by simply becoming your own best-educated advocate. Eating cruciferous vegetables (e.g., broccoli, cauliflower, kohlrabi, etc.) may help you decrease your risk of breast cancer by altering how your body metabolizes estrogen. Decreasing saturated fat intake (fat that's solid at room temperature) and exercising regularly may also be helpful.

The point here is that **you can take charge of your health better than anyone else.** This doesn't mean you run immediately to a dietician or a physical trainer. It does mean that you instead learn what's feasible for you to do for yourself. One trap to avoid is trying to make radical changes overnight. These are seldom sustainable, and truly healthy change must create a new lifestyle for you that you can follow consistently. The authors have found that the most lasting changes come about gradually and are implemented slowly, step-by-step, based on realistic expectations. As physicians and patients ourselves, we know what it means to have to make meaningful changes, and we will help you identify what your problems are, as well as how you can effectively change them. In the second part of this book, we provide a systematic program to help you define and reach your health goals. We also define the specific tests you should take to determine and modify your risk for diseases.

Now that we've talked a bit about women, let's talk a little about men. The most common cancer in men is prostate cancer, and it is the second leading cause of cancer mortality, after lung cancer, among men in the United States. This disease disproportionately affects African American men. A man's risk for developing prostate cancer increases as his age does, according to the following general rule: 50 percent risk at fifty years old, 60 percent at sixty years old, 70 percent at seventy years old, and so forth. The older one gets, however, the less aggressive the cancer is likely to be, and the less likely it is that a man will die from the prostate cancer itself versus some other cause.

The incidence of prostate cancer is 60 percent higher in African American men than it is in white men. Compared to Asian/Pacific Islanders, African American men are three times more likely to get prostate cancer and six times more likely to die from it. A review of fourteen case-controlled studies and nine cohort studies concluded that dairy intake "is one of the most consistent dietary predictors for prostate cancer in the published literature." Data from the Physicians' Health Study, in which diet and prostate cancer incidence were documented in 20,885 male physicians for eleven years, showed that those who consumed more than 2.5 servings of dairy products per day had a 34 percent greater risk of getting prostate cancer compared to those who consumed 0.5 servings per day. While various races may exhibit increased risk of some diseases, likely due to some genetic predisposition, what the authors have discovered is that modifying dietary habits significantly reduces risk of prostate cancer.

Again, what's crucial to understand is that you cannot change your genes, but you can change your diet and your lifestyle. What can people do if they're told that they have a genetic risk? After all, you cannot alter your genes. Will you get a radical mastectomy if you have the gene for breast cancer? Will you get a radical prostatectomy if you're at increased genetic risk of prostate cancer? Possibly. But much less risky and potentially more beneficial is to change your diet and lifestyle.

Improve Your Health

If you're in a high-risk category because of your lifestyle or exposure to environmental toxins, or if you have a family member (grandparent, uncle, aunt, mother, father, sister, or brother) with a major health condition, such as cardiovascular disease, your recommendations for testing are different (tables 2.2 and 2.3).

Table 2.2. Abbreviated List of Risk Factors for Diseases.

Family History	Lifestyle
Cancer (eg, colorectal, breast, cervical)	Lack of exercise
Diabetes	Excess weight
Cardiovascular Disease	Chronic stress
Dementia	Profession (eg, roofers, office workers, graveyard shift)
Autoimmune diseases	**Environmental Toxins**
	Toxic Metals

Table 2.3. Routine Physical exams and Tests for High-Risk Patients

Age	Physical Exams and Tests

18-39	• **Women and Men:**
	  ✓ Monthly: skin check (moles and birthmarks)
	  ✓ Annually: Dental exam and cleaning, blood pressure (can be done at most local drug stores for free), skin check (moles and birthmarks)
	  ✓ **Family history of heart disease:** Twice during your thirties: lipid panel (cholesterols, triglycerides), inflammatory markers (C-reactive protein, ferritin, fibrinogen), lipid peroxides, intracellular magnesium, fasting insulin, homocysteine
	  ✓ **Family history of obesity or diabetes:** Twice during your twenties and three times during your thirties: lipid panel (cholesterols, triglycerides), inflammatory markers (C-reactive protein, ferritin, fibrinogen), lipid peroxides, intracellular magnesium, fasting insulin, homocysteine, fasting blood glucose.
	• **Women, family history of any females cancers (breast, cervical, ovarian):**
	  ✓ Monthly: self breast exam
	  ✓ Once in early 20s: urinary 2-16 hydroxyestrogen ratio, serum 8-Hydroxy-2-deoxyguanosine (marker for free radical damage to DNA)
	  ✓ At 25 years old: mammogram
	  ✓ Annually: pelvic exam and pap smear
	• **Men with family history of prostate cancer:**
	  • Monthly: monthly self testicular exam
	  • At 30 years old, then every three years: PSA test

40-65	• **Women and Men:**
	  ✓ Monthly: skin check (moles and birthmarks)
	  ✓ Annually: dental exam and cleaning every year, blood pressure (can be done for free at most drug stores), cholesterol (if you have a previous abnormal test), rectal exam and stool guiac test for colorectal cancer screening
	  ✓ Every one to five years: physical exam
	  ✓ Every two years: eye exam after age of 40, including a check for glaucoma.
	  ✓ Every three years: fasting blood glucose to screen for diabetes
	  ✓ Every three to five years: flexible sigmoidoscopy beginning at age 50
	  ✓ Every five years: cholesterol (if elevated, check yearly)
	  ✓ At 40 years old: lean body mass measurement, then every 5 years
	• **Women:** monthly self breast exam; yearly pelvic exam and pap smear; mammogram every 1 to 2 years once over the age of 40 and yearly after age of 50; baseline bone density scan at age 60
	• **Men:** yearly rectal exam after age of 50; yearly PSA blood test for prostate cancer risk after 50; baseline bone density scan at age 60

Over the age of 65	• **Women and Men:**
	  ✓ Monthly: Skin check (moles and birthmarks) monthly self exams
	  ✓ Annually: Dental exam and cleaning, hearing test, blood

	pressure (can be done for free at most drug stores), physical exam, rectal exam and stool guiac test to screen for colorectal cancer ✓ Every two years: eye exam, including check for glaucoma ✓ Every three years: fasting blood glucose to screen for diabetes ✓ Every three to five years: cholesterol (if normal, more frequently if abnormal), flexible sigmoidoscopy to screen for polyps and colorectal cancer (or colonoscopy every 10 years) • **Women:** monthly self breast exam; pelvic exam and pap smear every 1 to 3 years; mammogram yearly • **Men:** yearly rectal exam and PSA test to screen for prostrate cancer

*If moles or birthmarks are changing in color or size, see a Dermatologist.

Problems essentially become challenges that you can use to your advantage. What we're explaining in this book is that every seeming obstacle is an opportunity to improve yourself. The way you think about yourself and health problems become exceedingly important. The major point here is that you are in charge of your health and healthcare, even to the point of being able to order your own laboratory tests. You are your best advocate. Later in this book, we list specific medical tests that you may order directly. Second, doctors who tell you something is genetic, or who say there's nothing more that you can do, are in most cases doing you a disservice. It's imperative for your health to ignore the notion of a fatalistic, predetermined outcome that has been imposed on you. Sometimes the almost direst diagnosis by a physician can be the most easily treated problem. But once again, it depends on you—and your willingness to be your own best advocate.

Chapter 3:
Components of Health

The fact that you're reading this book means that you might be interested in health. But what is health? Everybody talks about health, certainly about "better health" and "improved health," but what exactly does it mean to be healthy?

Health is not merely the absence of disease. In our opinion, someone with terminal cancer can still be healthy. An often-overlooked component of health is realism. That is, being realistic about who you are, where you're at in your life, and where you're headed. In short, what we're saying is that health is not defined by your state of body or mind, but by your ability to do something for yourself at any given point in your life. Also, health entails a mindset that allows you to accept new paradigms of science, nutrition, and lifestyle, incorporating them into your daily routines in such a way that they make you feel better physically and happier and more content emotionally.

Health is a mindset of incorporating the past with the present to invent a new future. Health is the interaction among seven components: physical, intellectual, emotional, spiritual, financial, social, and professional.

As complicated as medicine has made the diagnosis of diseases, there really are few underlying causes of disease. Health practitioners divide the body into nine different systems: immune, cardiovascular, neurological, digestive, endocrine, excretory, musculoskeletal, reproductive, and respiratory. You do not need to know all the technical details of each of these systems. What is important is understanding a couple of basic concepts of how the different systems interrelate and how you can affect them. This will allow you to understand better why the authors have structured their health recommendations, which they created based on the most important indicators of health.

Physical: Health Starts in the Gut

Unbeknownst to most allopathic physicians, of primary importance to overall health is the health of the digestive system. In this book, we call it "gut health." Recently, Dr. Pieczenik was reacquainted with a physician who was Dr. Pieczenik's neurology supervisor when Dr. Pieczenik was a fourth-year medical student. Dr. Pieczenik had a discussion with this neurologist, who became Chief Neurologist of a major regional medical center.

Dr. Pieczenik asked this esteemed mentor what had been accomplished in the last thirty years in neurology, since Dr. Pieczenik had been a medical student. The response was that there were basically ten major neurological diseases, which could be diagnosed with the extensive and highly expensive technology of MRIs, CT scans, and invasive procedures. These technologies had substituted for the basic physical examinations in neurology, which were overall quite sensitive and specific, compared to the new technologies. However, the new technology allowed physicians to spend less time with their patients and rely on technology instead of their clinical medicine skills. In effect, Dr. Pieczenik's mentor admitted that he had become a manager of technology more so than a direct clinician.

In fact, some specialists now, such as neurologists, may be able to work for several days without ever touching a patient. Allopathic medical students today, including Dr. Pieczenik's daughter, who is a fourth-year medical student at a major New York City medical school, are rarely taught physical diagnosis. They spend most of their time being patient administrators and managers of technology.

The Chief Neurologist took great pride in telling Dr. Pieczenik that the greatest development in recent years in treatments for neurological diseases, such as Multiple Sclerosis, was basically sophisticated anti-inflammatory agents. When Dr. Pieczenik asked this neurologist why he didn't use natural methods, the neurologist said that there was not sufficient research to prove their effectiveness.

Dr. Pieczenik asked, "How can you know this? There are more than six million articles in the National Library of Medicine's database. Have you looked at all the research on turmeric, for example?" The neurologist replied that he was not aware of all these citations, nor had he ever looked at the studies on turmeric.

> **Individual Health Profile: Sally**
>
> Sally was a 42 year old woman who worked as an attorney for a prestigious law firm. At about the age of 38 she began to suffer from depression and fatigue. She was prescribed the typical rounds of antidepressant medications, which helped to some degree, but she continued to feel worse as time went on. She consulted with Dr. Neustadt, who helped her decrease her stress and improve her diet to help promote her health. The biochemical impact of the stress was detected by running tests that showed depletions in amino acids, vitamins and minerals, as well as multiple food allergies.
>
> **Health Lesson:** Stress has a direct correlation to biochemical deficiencies and is an important underlying cause of many conditions. Over several months her energy and mood improved and she felt a renewed sense of well-being and purpose, and she discontinued her antidepressant medications.

More importantly, Dr. Pieczenik asked him, "Where is the center of the immune system?"

The neurologist replied, "In the lymphatics." The lymphatics technically are simply the tubes in the body that drain into lymph nodes. You may be able to feel your lymph nodes in your armpits, in your neck and in your groin. They frequently become enlarged when you're sick.

The neurologist was flat-out wrong. Approximately 80 percent of all immune proteins are produced in the gut.[11] The immune tissue in the gut is called gut-associated lymph tissue (GALT) and is the largest immune organ in the body.[12] This makes sense when you begin thinking functionally instead of simply memorizing facts. What's the role of the immune system? Very simply, it protects you from the outside world—bacteria, viruses, and parasites. What part of your body is most exposed to the outside world? Most people intuitively would say their skin, but in fact it's your intestines (stomach, small and large intestines). The intestines have a surface area that's 3,229 to 4,306 square feet, which is 20 percent of a football field![13] (An American football field has a surface area of 21,600 square feet.)

Technically, your intestines are outside the body. They form a hollow tube from mouth to anus. When you put food or drink in your mouth, it doesn't actually enter your body until it is absorbed through the cells lining your gut. Your intestines' exposure to the outside world and all its dangerous microbes is awesome when you think that every day the average person consumes three to five pounds of food.[13] And every piece of food contains potentially millions of organisms, both harmful and beneficial.

Even when someone is eating an optimal diet, he may not be digesting and assimilating the nutrients properly. There are three major reasons for this. His digestion may not be functioning properly; he may have food intolerances that cause chronic immune activation in the gut;[14-16] or he may have bacterial or fungal infections in the gut, called *intestinal dysbiosis*.[14, 17] Each of these situations can occur individually or together, and all result in putting one at risk for decreased ability to absorb nutrients.

Digestion involves the breakdown of large molecules into smaller, readily absorbed molecules. While some digestion begins with the production of enzymes in the mouth, the stomach is where the process of digestion really gets under way. Cells in the stomach excrete specific enzymes to break apart fats, starches, and proteins. The enzymes, however, are inactive and must be activated by stomach acid. When someone produces enough stomach acid, proper digestion in the stomach occurs. But many people don't produce enough stomach acid. Low stomach acid production is called *hypochlorhydria,* and when no stomach acid is produced, it's called *achlorhydria*. Decreased stomach acid production occurs from aging, caffeine, overeating, stress, medications (especially those that block the production or excretion of stomach acid, such as Protonix, Tagamet, Pepcid, Axid, Zantac, Prevacid, Prilosec, Aciphex, Nexium), alcohol, and stomach surgeries that destroy the acid-producing cells.

Many people produce less stomach acid as they age, and it's been estimated that 10–21 percent of people sixty to sixty-nine years old, 31 percent of those seventy to seventy-nine years old, and 37 percent of those above the age of eighty have hypochlorhydria or achlorhydria, and this rate may be higher in people with autoimmune conditions.[18, 19] One question posed to patients to screen for their risk of low stomach acid is, "Do you feel fuller sooner than you used to, and stay full longer than you used to when you eat?" If the answer is yes, it may be that they have low stomach acid, since decreased stomach acid increases the amount of time food sits in the stomach before passing into the small intestines. When stomach acid is low, vitamins and minerals may not be efficiently released from the food that contains them.

This may result in decreased availability of nutrients for absorption and nutritional deficiencies. People with low stomach acid have been shown to be at increased risk for vitamin and mineral deficiencies.[20-24] Symptoms of low stomach acid production include bloating or distension after eating, diarrhea or constipation, flatulence after a meal, hair loss in women, heartburn, indigestion, malaise, and prolonged sense of fullness after eating.[24, 25] Additionally, the risk of hip fracture increases by 22 percent after one year and nearly 60 percent after four years in people taking acid-blocking medications, as compared to people not taking them.[26]

Stomach acid plays two other important roles. It acts to sterilize food and signals the lower esophageal sphincter (the muscle separating the esophagus from the stomach) to close.[27-29] The gut normally contains about four hundred different species of bacteria, which are required for normal digestion and absorption of nutrients.[30, 31] It has been estimated that there are more bacterial cells in the gut than all the cells in the body combined.[32] These beneficial bacteria are required for normal digestion and absorption of nutrients. When inadequate sterilization of food occurs, however, pathogenic (bad) bacteria, viruses, and fungi can pass into the small intestines. This disrupts the healthy ecology in the gut and alters the delicate balance between healthy and unhealthy microbes.

This imbalance in intestinal flora is called *dysbiosis*, and it can occur with the overgrowth of pathogenic bacteria and/or fungus. Symptoms of intestinal dysbiosis include abdominal gas and bloating, postnasal drip, "brain fog" (feeling like you're just not mentally sharp), and sugar cravings.[33] Abdominal gas and bloating are caused by fermentation of food by the bacteria and fungus, which causes the production of gas, such as methane. Postnasal drip is caused by immune system activation by bacteria and fungi. Sugar is the preferred energy source for the fungi, which can lead to sugar cravings. Bacteria and fungi secrete their own waste products, such as ammonia, that can enter the bloodstream, cross into the brain, and cause brain fog. Additionally, intestinal bacterial overgrowth is now understood to be a risk factor for developing gastroesophageal reflux disorder (GERD).[34]

Simple tests can detect pathogenic intestinal bacteria and fungi (yeast). One test evaluates acids in your urine that are produced specifically by intestinal bacteria and yeast. These acids enter the bloodstream from the intestines, are filtered by the kidneys, and are then excreted in the urine. They include d-arabinitol, p-hydroxybenzoate, indican, tricarballylate and dihydroxyphenylpropionate.[33] Stool tests can also be run to detect stomach and intestinal infections, including bacteria, yeast, and parasites.

When low stomach acid production decreases the ability of the lower esophageal sphincter to close, the result is that the acid produced in the stomach can reflux up into the esophagus and cause symptoms of GERD.[35] The typical medical response to gastric reflux, which can cause burning, coughing, and asthma-like symptoms, is to prescribe acid-blocking medications.

However, the actual cause in many people is too little acid, not too much acid.[35] Decreased acid production can occur as a result of decreased histidine, an amino acid that is required for acid secretion.[36] This amino acid is tested as part of an amino acid blood panel, which may diagnose the underlying cause in some patients. Stomach acid production can also be tested by using a meter called a Heidelburg pH capsule test. Providing histidine to people with low stomach acid can improve their stomach acid production. Low stomach acid can also occur from infections, such as *Helicobacter pylori* (*H. pylori*), in the stomach.[35] Additionally, when people have low stomach acid production, some doctors provide hydrochloric acid capsules for people to take with meals, which helps improve their digestion and eliminate GERD. However, there are some instances when people should not supplement with acid pills, and the authors of this book strongly advise people against supplementing with hydrochloric acid unless under the care of a doctor.

Food intolerances can also cause decreased absorption of nutrients by creating chronic inflammation in the intestines. Eighty percent of the immune system is clustered around the intestines.[11] When people repeatedly consume food that causes an immune activation in the gut, it creates intestinal irritation.[37] Over time, the cells lining the intestines become damaged. This can create malabsorption, with decreased ability to assimilate nutrients from food. An extreme example of this is Celiac disease. Intolerance to wheat, rye, barley, and oats characterizes this disease. The immune system actually reacts to gluten contained in these foods. This causes intestinal inflammation and destruction of the cells lining the intestines. Celiac disease has wide-ranging symptoms, including fatigue, anemia, joint pain, depression, loss of balance, and malnutrition.[38, 39]

More frequently, people will react to foods that they crave, such as milk and eggs, which can be detected through a special blood test. This blood test is called an IgG food intolerance test, and people with rheumatoid arthritis, eczema, and other conditions have been shown to have elevated IgG antibodies to foods.[40, 41] IgG is a protein produced by the immune system. Most doctors only test for IgE-mediated allergies, which are also called "immediate hypersensitivity reactions." An IgE-mediated immune response is responsible for the life-threatening reaction some people have to bee stings or peanuts. IgG, on the other hand, is a delayed-type hypersensitivity reaction that, as the name implies, is not immediately apparent.[42] People who test negative on an IgE test can be positive on an IgG test.[43]

IgG reactions may take hours or days to appear, and symptoms can include postnasal drip, gas and bloating, difficulty losing weight, joint aches, eczema, fatigue, and others. Food intolerances can cause these diverse symptoms for various reasons. Similar to bacterial and fungal dysbiosis, the immune system activation caused by food intolerances can cause postnasal drip. Gas and bloating are a result of incomplete digestion of food and the resultant fermentation of these food particles by bacteria in the intestines. Difficulty losing weight may result from an increased cortisol response by the body due to the continual stress placed on the immune system. When cortisol is chronically elevated, it causes an accumulation of abdominal fat.

The explanation for eczema and joint pain is a little more complicated. When the immune system in the intestines is activated, the antibody-antigen complexes enter the bloodstream. An antibody is the protein produced by the immune system, such as IgG, and an antigen is the molecule against which the immune system is reacting, such as a protein in milk. These antibody-antigen complexes travel from the intestines to the liver, where they are broken down for elimination by the body. This process is like a conveyor belt, whereby the antibody-antigen complexes are delivered to the liver for processing, but the amount of complexes delivered to the liver over time can overwhelm the liver's ability to detoxify them.

When this occurs, the complexes pass through the liver and enter the systemic circulation. Like bits of sand in a river, these complexes can settle out of the bloodstream, where the flow of blood slows down. This occurs in the skin and joints. When these complexes are deposited in skin and joints, they act as irritants that can create local immune system activation and produce such symptoms as joint pain and eczema. The joint pain will often be *migratory*, meaning different joints will be affected at different times.

Chronic stress predisposes people to low stomach acid production and food intolerances. This is because stress stimulates the release of cortisol, norepinephrine, and epinephrine. These are part of the flight-or-flight response to stress. The analogy that's often used to teach this concept to medical student is to imagine that you're being chased by a tiger. The body has two responses. It either flees or battles it out. In either case, cortisol and epinephrine are secreted to prepare people for action. They increase blood flow to skeletal muscles and decrease it to the intestines. These hormones also increase heart rate and alter blood flow in the brain. By shifting blood flow away from the intestines and to the muscles, digestion decreases. This can also cause damage to the cells lining the intestines and create a "hyperpermeable gut." When digestion decreases, it allows larger food particles to enter the small intestines, where food is absorbed through the lining of the gut and into the body. The larger food particles, combined with the damaged lining of the gut, can activate the immune system and create food intolerances.

As you now understand, many health complaints are directly related to and caused by an unhealthy intestinal tract. Identifying any food allergies and intestinal infections are crucial to healing the gut. The goal is remove the things (e.g., aggravating foods and infections) that are causing the problems, and then initiate a gut-repair protocol using specific nutrients to heal the gut. One key nutrient is L-Glutamine, an amino acid that is an energy source for cells in your digestive tract. This provides nutrition to the gut to help the cells heal. Herbs that soothe the gut are also sometimes used. What's crucial in many cases is also reducing stress, which is discussed in this next section.

Mental: Stress, Stress, Stress

The importance of stress in overall health cannot be overemphasized. Many chronic diseases are directly related to and result from high levels of chronic stress. Stress comes in two basic forms—emotional and physical. In today's society, people are overwhelmingly burdened with both types of stress. They spend longer hours driving or stuck in traffic; spend more time working; spend twenty-four hours a day connected to their cell phones, Blackberries, and other wireless devices; feel burdened by the physical, emotional, and financial demands of having a family; and are concerned with national and international political situations. All these factors conspire to create a constant state of agitation in people.

Humans were not designed to endure this level of constant stress. The nervous system is primarily responsible for handling this stress. There are two components of the nervous system: the parasympathetic and the sympathetic nervous systems. The parasympathetic nervous system is activated during rest, and it is sometimes called *rest and digest*. When the parasympathetic arm of the nervous system is activated, it shuttles blood to the intestines for better digestion and absorption of nutrients.

Opposing the parasympathetic nervous system is the sympathetic nervous system, also called the fight-or-flight response. The sympathetic nervous system causes a secretion of stress hormones, including epinephrine and cortisol, and shuttles blood away from the intestines and to large muscles. Why? Because this part of the nervous system is there to save you from perceived danger. The body's automatic response is to get ready to either fight or run away.

When you are continually in a fight-or-flight situation, the effect on the organ systems is incredibly detrimental. Why? It decreases your production of stomach acid and your ability to digest and absorb nutrients. It increases your risk for food allergies and intestinal infections. It causes depletions of amino acid, as well as vitamins and minerals. It causes increased free radical damage, decreased ability to regulate blood sugar, damage to the memory centers in your brain, and alterations in your immune function. It creates a situation that damages mitochondria (the energy producing part of our cells) and promotes disease. Chronic stress is a major contributing factor to the development and progression of osteoporosis, dementia, cardiovascular disease, obesity, and cancer.

Toxins: It's a Toxic World, after All

When Dr. Neustadt was a boy living in Southern California, he would go twice a year to Disneyland to celebrate his and his brother's birthdays. He enjoyed the "It's a Small World" ride. For those readers who don't know this ride, imagine yourself in a small boat traveling slowly down a canal. On either side are animated characters singing the theme song in different languages.

As time goes on, the world indeed has become smaller. Economic and technological globalization has resulted in a veritable explosion of toxic chemicals being produced and transported around the world. Modern society has developed an extensive array of synthetic chemicals over the last several decades—chemicals to control disease, increase food production, and to provide convenience in our daily lives. While the standard use in our society of over seventy-five thousand different chemical compounds has offered added convenience and productivity in our lives, it has also come at a tremendous price.

Toxic Chemicals

It has been estimated that as much as ten million (yes, *million!*) pounds of mercury are released into the atmosphere every year from burning coal and natural gas, and refining petroleum products. This metal is highly toxic to the nervous system and can travel for hundreds or even thousands of miles on wind currents, depositing far from its source. Aside from industrial sources, common sources of mercury toxicity occur in fish and dental fillings. The fish that contain the highest concentrations of mercury are warm-water fish, such as tuna and yellowtail.

Children are especially susceptible to mercury and other toxicities. Mercury exposure can impair children's memories, attention, and language abilities, as well as interfere with fine motor and visual spatial skills. And in a pregnant woman, mercury can cross the placenta and accumulate in her unborn child. Mercury toxicity can create many symptoms (table 3.1).

Table 3.1. Symptoms of Mercury Toxicity	
Neurological	**Non-Neurological**
Ataxia	Alopecia totalis (complete loss of hair)
Chorea	Autoimmune disease
Blindness	Fatigue
Depression	Hypersalivation
Drowsiness	Keratosis
Excitability	Melanosis (darkening of skin)
Fearfulness/anxiety	Recurrent infections
Insomnia	Ulcers
Irritability	
Low intelligence quotient (IQ)	
Memory loss	
Mental retardation	
Parasthesias (change in sensations)	
Quarreling	
Restlessness	
Temper outbursts	
Tremors	

Dietary supplements are also a source of potential toxic metals contamination. The medical literature supports using nutraceuticals for many conditions, including taking iron to correct iron deficiency anemia, taking alpha lipoic acid to reverse diabetic peripheral neuropathy, coenzyme Q10 for cardiomyopathy, magnesium for muscle cramps, and L-carnitine for physical and mental fatigue.

However, many of the dietary supplements sold in health food stores and drugstores carry some serious potential problems. The dietary supplement industry is regulated by the FDA, under the Dietary Supplement Health and Education Act (DSHEA) passed in 1994.

When it was enacted, DSHEA classified dietary supplements as foods, not food additives, which exempted them from having to prove their safety or efficacy.

The first problem is that you may not actually be getting in the bottle what's on the label. Manufacturers are not required to test products going to market to ensure that they actually contain the ingredients they claim. In one study of twenty-four ginseng products, one-third of the products contained no active ingredients at all.

The second problem is toxic metals. A survey of dietary supplements produced in South Asia and sold in twenty stores in the Boston area in 2006 revealed that 20 percent of the dietary supplements contained heavy metals. Of those with heavy metals, thirteen contained toxic levels of lead, six tested positive for arsenic, and six contained mercury. A 2002 case report documented lead poisoning in a forty-one-year-old man, resulting from a dietary supplement containing herbs from India. This man complained of malaise, weakness, abdominal pain, and weight loss. His blood tested high for lead. Analysis of the dietary supplements revealed high concentrations of lead.

Another case report from 2002 described arsenic toxicity in a thirty-nine-year-old woman taking the dietary supplement Chitosan*, which is derived from chitin found in shellfish. It is used to help people lose weight by blocking the absorption and storage of fat. The woman reported to the emergency room complaining of fatigue, headache, and weakness for the past six months. For a year, she had been taking six capsules daily of the "fat blocker" pills. A twenty-four-hour urine collection revealed extremely elevated arsenic. Analysis of the pills showed high levels of arsenic, and shellfish are known to store arsenic.

Aside from the aforementioned potential dangers, many people are simply wasting their money on dietary supplements that do not contain ingredients the body can even use. The body does not absorb all forms of nutrients to the same degree. If your multivitamin contains magnesium in its oxide form, which is commonly used because it's less expensive to manufacture, you are only absorbing about 2 percent of what's actually in a pill. For example if the label states that the dietary supplement contains 100 mg magnesium as magnesium oxide, you're only effectively absorbing 2 mg into your body. In contrast, the most absorbable form of minerals, of which magnesium is one, is the amino acid chelated form. Look for magnesium amino acid chelate on the list of ingredients.

In conclusion, its buyer beware. Many people are purchasing dietary supplements without truly understanding what they're buying. First, look at the label closely and make sure that it reads "purity and potency guaranteed" or "tested for purity and potency." Assume all products are contaminated and don't contain the amount of nutrients in the bottle that is listed on the label, unless otherwise stated on the bottle that they've been tested for purity and potency. Next, ask the sales staff what the most absorbable forms of nutrients are, and the amounts that are most appropriate for a given dietary supplement. If they don't know, you may find good information on the internet or by discussing this with your doctor.

Pesticides are also a major source of concern. A complete review of all pesticides is beyond the scope of this book. However, the authors would like to give you a taste of the scope of the problem. Each year in America, we use over 2.2 billion pounds of pesticides, or 8 pounds for every man woman and child in the country. Pesticides are toxic substances deliberately added to our environment to kill living things. This includes substances that kill weeds (herbicides), insects (insecticides), and fungus (fungicides).

The humble little blueberry, rich in flavor and healthy antioxidants, is a poster child for pesticides in our food system. On more than sixty thousand acres of cropland, Maine produces 25 percent of all blueberries in North America. Although blueberries in Maine grow wild, as their economic importance has increased, farmers have come to rely on toxic pesticides to increase production. Large-scale blueberry monoculture requires significant pest control measures to protect the commodity. The Maine Board of Pesticides Control (BPC) found that the blueberry industry used the following fifteen trade-name pesticides (active ingredient in parentheses):

- Benlate (Benomyl)—fungicide
- (Captan)—fungicide
- (Diazinon ag)—insecticide
- Elevate (Fenhexamid)—fungicide
- Funginex (Triforine)—fungicide
- Gramoxone (Paraquat)—herbicide
- Guthion (Azinphos-methyl)—insecticide
- Imidan (Phosmet)—insecticide
- Orbit (Propiconazole)—fungicide
- Poast (Sethoxydim)—herbicide
- Roundup (Glyphosate)—herbicide
- Select (Clethodim)—herbicide
- Sencor (Metribuzin)—herbicide
- Thiodan (Endosulfan)—insecticide
- Velpar (Hexazinone)—herbicide

In addition to these fifteen pesticides, the University of Maine Cooperative Extension recommends nine fungicides for use on blueberry crops. Of those:

- 67 percent (six) are possible carcinogens according to the EPA

- 44 percent (four) cause reproductive or developmental effects or are endocrine disruptors
- 33 percent (three) are moderately to highly toxic through acute exposures

Of the ten insecticides recommended for use on blueberry crops:
- 33 percent (three) are possible carcinogens according to the EPA
- 40 percent (four) cause reproductive or developmental effects or are endocrine disruptors
- 60 percent (six) are moderately to highly toxic through acute exposures

Of the seven herbicides recommended for use on blueberry crops:
- 14 percent (one) is a known carcinogen according to the EPA
- 14 percent (one) causes reproductive or developmental effects
- 29 percent (two) are moderately to highly toxic through acute exposure

Of the 26 active ingredients for use by the blueberry industry:
- 62 percent (sixteen) are moderately to very highly toxic to aquatic life
- 65 percent (seventeen) cause chronic problems in aquatic life

Toxic Drift

Toxic Drift is the movement of pesticides (and other chemicals) in the air, away from the area where they are applied. Pesticide drift can cause many problems for both humans and the environment. Since 2002, at least ten toxic drift complaints have been reported to the BPC. These reports include complaints of applicators spraying in extremely windy conditions, organic blueberry fields being contaminated by pesticide drift, and residents being hit directly by spray.

These reports signify that people are not only expressing concerns for their health, but also fearing that pesticide drift is contaminating their property. Since 1999, the BPC has worked to monitor residues from blueberry pesticide drift. In 2001, they reported that pesticides traveled nearly one mile from their site of application. And there is an entire category of chemicals that are known or suspected endocrine disruptors. These chemicals can interfere with the human hormonal system, particularly the thyroid gland. During pregnancy, the hormones released by the thyroid are vital for normal development of the fetus's brain.

Unfortunately, some of these chemicals make good flame retardants and have been widely used in everything from upholstery to televisions to children's clothing. Studies have found them in high levels in household dust, as well as in breast milk. Two categories of these flame retardants have been banned in Europe and are starting to be banned by different states in the United States.

Other chemicals, called plasticizers, are just now coming onto the radar screen as possible sources of health problems. One of them, bisphenol A, is found in pacifiers, baby bottles, and dental sealant used to prevent cavities in children. In 2007, California banned all bisphenol A from children's products, citing serious health concern. Research on bisphenol A has shown that it can affect both the reproductive and neurological system, and that it appears to accumulate at higher concentrations around the fetus—in the umbilical cord and amniotic fluid—than in the mother's blood.

In conclusion, never have so many toxins been produced and disseminated so widely in so many products. Our world has truly become a small world of toxins. Lest you become too fearful, the authors just want to say that you have to be very careful about where your products come from, whether they're organic or not.

But the problem of toxic drift is much more serious and global. A sweeping six-year U.S. Environmental Protection Agency (EPA) study titled "Western Airborne Contaminants Assessment Project" was released in early 2008. It concluded that pesticides, heavy metals, and other airborne contaminants are raining down on national parks across the West and Alaska, turning up at sometimes dangerously high levels in lakes, plants, and fish. It found more than seventy different contaminants in twenty national parks, in such pristine areas as Denali National Park in Alaska, Glacier National Park in Montana, Big Bend National Park in Texas, and Yosemite National Park in California.

The researchers found elevated levels of mercury, PCB, and DDT, pesticides that were banned in the United States more than twenty years ago. These contaminants, which cause neurological damage, impair the immune system, and can cause sterility, accumulate in fish. Contaminants that accumulated in fish exceeded human consumption thresholds at the eight parks.

Where are these toxins coming from? Much of the contamination is thought to have come from overseas—traveling global air currents from Europe and Asia. But many are also drifting on air currents from farmland in the United States, where tons of pesticides are applied each year to croplands.

Toxic Water

The most basic necessity of life besides air is water. Approximately 75 percent of the body is composed of water. Every biochemical reaction in the body occurs in an aqueous environment. So what is the problem with water? Here it is.

Our use of manmade chemicals has become so extreme that we can now find traces of these low-level toxins in virtually every public water supply in the world. A report by the Ralph Nader Study Group, after reviewing over ten thousand documents acquired through the Freedom of Information Act, stated, "U.S. drinking water contains more than 2,100 toxic chemicals that can cause cancer."

The Federal Council on Environmental Quality reports that "up to two-thirds of all cancers may be attributed to these low level toxins," and that "once contaminated, our groundwater will remain so for tens of thousands of years."

Our tendency is to blame it on the big factories upstream. And while industry has certainly played its part in our water contamination problems, consumers of a vast array of products are also to blame. The majority of the contaminants found in our drinking water can be traced back to improper or excessive use of ordinary compounds like lawn chemicals, gasoline, cleaning products and even prescription drugs.

Everything that goes down the drain, on our lawns, on our agricultural fields, or into the environment by any means, eventually winds up in the water we drink. Once we realize this, we begin to see just how fragile our water supplies really are.

Water Treatment Facilities Are Not Enough

Our municipal water treatment facilities are not designed or effective for removing these synthetic chemicals; they typically only consist of sand bed filtration and disinfection, much like a standard swimming pool filter.

A 1994 study of twenty-nine major U.S. cities by the Environmental Working Group found that all those cities had traces of at least one

47

weed killer in the drinking water. The report titled "Tap Water Blues" went on to say that "millions of Americans are routinely exposed to one or more pesticides in a single glass of tap water."

These first ever tap water testings found two or more pesticides in the drinking water of twenty-seven of the twenty-nine cities, three or more in twenty-four cities, four or more in twenty-one cities, five or more in eighteen cities, six or more in thirteen cities, and seven or more pesticides in the tap water of five cities. In Fort Wayne, Indiana, nine different pesticides were found in a single glass of tap water.

As a startling side note, it was reported that in these twenty-nine cities, forty-five thousand infants drank formula mixed with tap water containing weed killers, and that "over half of these infants were swallowing four to nine chemicals in every bottle."

The tragic health effects of consuming these highly toxic chemicals are magnified many times over for small children because their systems are more sensitive and still developing. Small children also consume a much larger volume of fluids per pound of body weight, and therefore get a bigger dose, yet none of these factors are considered when the EPA's maximum contaminant levels are set.

The National Academy of Sciences issued a report in 1993 on this subject, stating that "children are not little adults, their bodies are less developed and incapable of detoxifying certain harmful compounds."

Another major flaw in the estimated risks of chemicals in our drinking water is the false assumption that only one chemical is being consumed. The regulations are set based on what is assumed safe for a 175-pound adult drinking water with only that one chemical present; it does not take into account the combined toxicity of two or more chemicals.

In a 1995 Science Advisory Report to the EPA, it was stated that "when two or more of these contaminants combine in our water the potency may be increased by as much as one thousand times." Regardless of the differing opinions, it is safe to assume that there is no acceptable level for pesticides and weed killers in our drinking water.

Industrial solvents like TCE and benzene make their way into our water supplies from literally hundreds of sources. Airports and military bases degrease planes and engine parts with TCE, one of the most concentrated toxins in existence. One teaspoon of TCE will render over 250,000 gallons of water undrinkable, yet thousands of gallons are used in uncontained applications each day.

Perchlorethelyne, cyanide, and benzene are used in such common industries as dry cleaning, car washes, and photo processing, much of which ends up going down someone's drain and into our water supplies. It has been shown that areas with the highest levels of these carcinogens in their water supplies also have the highest incidence of cancer.

Chapter 4:
Routes of Detoxification

Please do not get overwhelmed by the information we have just presented to you. Even though you're surrounded by toxins, both inside and outside your body, you nevertheless can manage your exposure to these toxins as well as promote your own internal detoxification capability.

The human body's main routes of eliminating wastes and poisons are via the lymphatic, digestive, and urinary systems. Secondary routes of elimination include the skin and lungs. A foul odor on the breath or recurrent skin eruptions can be evidence of the lung and skin's attempt to assist overworked or weakened primary organs of elimination.

Let us first discuss the largest organ in the body. Do you know what that is? It's the skin. The skin makes up 12–15 percent of your body weight, with a surface area of about two square meters (21.5 square feet).

The skin separates and protects us from the outside world. But the skin is more than a simple barrier. It is a sense organ, an organ of detoxification, and a regulator of your internal temperature. Nerves in your skin detect pressure, pain, your location in space, and other sensations. Sweat eliminates toxins and cools you off when you're too hot. The inability to sweat upon exertion is an important symptom of Chronic Fatigue Syndrome, and it may indicate tired adrenal glands, also called *adrenal fatigue*. The adrenal glands are two glands that sit atop each of your kidneys and secrete many different hormones. Two of these, cortisol and epinephrine, are secreted during times of stress. During exertion, they help dilate blood vessels in your skin, which helps you begin to sweat and cool your body temperature when the sweat evaporates.

Therapies that promote perspiration assist the skin in moving wastes from the body. Hot baths, exercise, saunas, hydrotherapy, Epsom salt soaks, and any activity that enhances circulation in the skin and lymphatic channels can have a cleansing and stimulating effect. Most sauna detoxification programs use exercise, nutrients, and low-temperature long-duration heat exposure. These therapies increase the core body temperature, which has several stimulating effects. It increases the heart rate so that a larger volume of blood is filtered through the kidneys and liver in a shorter amount of time. It promotes immune function and the breakdown of toxins stored in fat cells. With an increase in respiration rate and with sweating, toxins are eliminated through the lungs and skin, respectively.

Improving elimination via the digestive system includes enhancing the activities of the liver's detoxification pathways, and promoting elimination via the stool. The liver is an amazing organ. It does more than four hundred different functions. One major role is to take toxins in the body and process them for elimination, either in the stool or the urine.

There are two basic phases of this process, appropriately called Phase I and Phase II. All steroid hormones, and most drugs, pesticides, and other environmental toxins, are inactivated and eliminated from the body by the excretory organs (kidneys, liver, lungs, skin, and bowels). The process serves to reduce the toxic load on the body and avoid internal toxin accumulation. It does this via the combined action of two separate but interrelated systems in the liver, called Phase I and Phase II detoxification.

The biochemical reactions in Phase I are driven by a family of enzymes known as cytochrome P450. They begin the process of detoxifying xenobiotics (substances produced outside the body and taken in either via the mouth, airway, or skin) such as petrochemical hydrocarbons and medications. They also detoxify endogenous substances (chemicals produced by the body), such as steroid hormones and other end products of metabolism, which would also be toxic if allowed to accumulate. In Phase I, the biochemical reaction involves the adding or exposing of a functional group to the toxic molecule. Like the different stations on an assembly line, in most cases the chemicals transformed in Phase I go directly into a Phase II reaction. However, the compound may be eliminated directly after the Phase I reaction.

The products generated from Phase I reactions are often highly reactive and unstable molecules that can cause local tissue damage. They are, in fact, often more toxic than the original compound. In order to be neutralized, they need to be shuttled through Phase II as quickly as possible.

After completing their transformation, the final products are then eliminated. In some cases, a toxin may be directly converted via Phase I or Phase II. Therefore, we return to the concept of balance. Both Phase I and Phase II pathways need to be in balance, relative to each other, for efficient and safe detoxification to proceed. If Phase II reactions are inhibited in some way, or if Phase I has been upregulated without a concomitant increase in Phase II, that optimal balance is compromised.

Molecules such as estrogen, Tylenol, cortisol, thyroid hormone, antidepressant drugs, and pain medications are all processed by these pathways. After they undergo their metabolic transformation, they are either packaged into bile and excreted with your feces, or sent to the kidneys for elimination in the urine.

Bile is a complex biochemical mixture, made continuously by the liver—500–1000 ml per day—passing down into the duodenum (small intestines) via the bile duct. On its way, bile enters the gallbladder, which stores the bile. Once you eat, the gallbladder contracts and empties its contents into the duodenum. Bile has two major functions. It emulsifies fat and increases its absorption, and it excretes the toxins processed by the liver into the intestines for elimination in the stool. Bile, which is 97 percent water, also contains bile salts composed of the amino acid taurine, as well as cholesterol, phospholipids, bile pigments, and electrolytes (minerals).

Many substances can affect how the detoxification process works. Nutrition plays a significant role. In general, the reactions involved in detoxification are driven by enzymes, which require cofactors, coenzymes, and other molecules provided through the diet. Provided by the diet, sulfur is one of these compounds used in the detoxification process. Drugs such as acetaminophen, which consume sulfur during detoxification, can decrease the function of this important system. Additionally, simply due to genetic individuality, one person may inherently be a more efficient detoxifier than someone else, even in the same family.

There are simple and convenient tests that can determine if your detoxification pathways are functioning optimally. Foods, herbs, and vitamins and minerals help the liver, lymphatic system, and hormonal and metabolic systems clear toxins from the body (table 4.1). Depending on the severity of the toxic load and the overall health of an individual, improving the vitality of the tissues can require several months to a year or more.

Table 4.1. Nutrients to Support Liver Detoxification Pathways[44-53]	
Vitamins	A (beta-carotene), B1 (thiamine), B2 (riboflavin), B3 (niacin), C (ascorbic acid), E, folic acid
Non-Vitamin Nutrients	Flavonoids, phospholipids, coenzyme Q10
Foods	Broccoli, cauliflower, kohlrabi, turmeric, chocolate, garlic, soy, grape skin
Minerals	Iron, selenium, zinc, copper, magnesium, manganese

Chapter 5:
Exercise

Exercise has consistently been shown in clinical trials to slow down the aging process, decrease risk of deadly diseases such as cancer, osteoporosis, infections, depression, and cardiovascular disease, among others. However, the caveat here is that exercise can only have these benefits when done appropriately. Exercising too frequently, too intensely, or using improper techniques can actually cause great harm.

The benefits of exercise are numerous. Resistance exercises (lifting weights or working against your own body weight) can prevent the onset of osteoporosis and strengthen muscles to decrease the risk of fractures in the elderly. Basic benefits of exercise reside in improved cardiovascular health. It improves blood flow, which in turns lowers the risk of hypertension, promotes immune function, and increases the "good cholesterol" (HDL cholesterol), while decreasing "bad cholesterol" (LDL cholesterol) and the risk of blood clots, as well as promoting sexual health by improving blood flow to the pelvis and the brain. Exercise also stimulates the release of endorphins, which are hormones that elevate mood. Exercise is associated with reduced risk of dementia.[54]

A 2007 study in the prestigious medical journal *Archives of Internal Medicine* concluded that consistent, moderate, and vigorous exercise may cut your risk of dying in half.[55] In a prospective study involving

252,925 subjects aged 50–71 years, results indicate that regular physical activity may be associated with reduced risk of mortality. Physical activity was assessed using questionnaires. Moderate activity entailed physical activity for at least twenty minutes per day on most days of the week, and vigorous exercise entailed exercise for at least thirty minutes per day, three times per week. Compared with being inactive, moderate activity decreased the risk of death by 27 percent and vigorous exercise with a 32 percent reduced mortality risk, respectively. Additionally, meeting both moderate activity and vigorous exercise recommendations was associated with a 50 percent reduced risk of mortality. This benefit even applied to people who smoked, were obese, or watched two or more hours of television or video per day.

But it's not just moderate to vigorous physical activity that can literally extend your life. The researchers also found that simply doing some physical activity reduced the risk of dying by 19 percent. Thus, the authors of this study conclude, "Following physical activity guidelines is associated with a reduced risk of death. Mortality benefit may also be achieved by engaging in less than recommended activity levels."

Most people tend to exercise in spurts. That is, they're weekend warriors. The authors believe very strongly that this exercise pattern is extremely dangerous. People go from a sedentary existence five days each week, and promise themselves that they can make up that deficit by overdoing it the other two days. The fact is that the only exercise pattern ever proven to provide consistent and dramatic health benefits is regular, routine exercising. Weekend warriors are putting their bodies under a tremendous amount of acute stress, which takes days to recover.

Equally important is a phenomenon the authors have noticed, but which has not yet been well documented in the medical literature, and that is an acute spasm of the bronchi, creating an abrupt oxygen deficiency that can lead to sudden death. For example, there's a case of a forty-two-year-old man who was exercising on a stationary bike and developed an acute constriction in his lungs. He had no history of allergies or asthma. He died suddenly. What the authors speculate happened is that he developed a predisposition to bronchospasms because of deficiencies in nutrients required to produce epinephrine. Epinephrine dilates the lungs and can be

Table 5.1. Benefits of Exercise[56]	
Resistance Exercise	Decreases insulin resistance Increases muscle Slows down the aging process Reduces blood pressure Improves bone health Aids in weight loss Reduces risk of falling
Aerobic	Decreases insulin resistance Elevates mood Increases "good cholesterol" Decreases "bad cholesterol" Aids in weight loss Improves cognitive function
Balance Training	Reduces risk of falling Improves mobility
Any Exercise	Improves insulin resistance Reduces risk of diabetes, cancer, and heart disease Reduces stress

depleted in people with mature onset asthma, such as Dr. Pieczenik. If the decrease in oxygen is sudden and severe, it can throw the heart into spasm, create an ischemia (low oxygen) situation in the heart muscle, and cause a heart attack.

The problem people have is starting and maintaining an effective and consistent exercise pattern. Many people create New Year's resolutions to exercise, perhaps even join a health club, and they exercise for a time. Invariably, most of these people stop exercising within a few months.

There are several reasons for this. One is that people simply get bored. Working out on the same machines and doing the same exercises in the same building, with the same people around you, becomes monotonous day after day. The next reason is that many people want immediate results, and they don't get them. There is a need for immediate self-gratification, which is not realistic. People often feel better quickly, but then plateau and do not see the incremental progress.

Additionally, many people are measuring the wrong criteria for improvement. Most people step on a scale and want to see pounds coming off. However, what they don't realize is that muscle weighs more than fat. So if you're working out and turning fat into muscle, the number on the scale won't necessarily come down. There are two much more sensitive indicators for progress. One is simply asking yourself how you feel and how your body feels. Do you feel that you move about easier when you walk, sit, or stand? Do you notice you're thinking more positively, or that normally stressful situations are affecting you less? Do your colleagues, family, or friends mention that they notice any differences in you?

The other sensitive indicator is what the authors like to call The Pants Test™. This test simply requires asking yourself if your pants are fitting looser, or if you're fastening your belt on a different notch. If the answer is yes, then you're making progress.

One issue is that if you're overweight, you likely have insulin resistance. Insulin resistance means that your body has difficulty burning sugars to create cellular energy. When this happens, instead of making energy, your body makes fat. When you start exercising, there may be a lag time in seeing physical results since your body will first work on correcting the hormonal imbalances to improve insulin resistance. Additionally, many people feel like they plateau and do not continue to see progress.

If this is the case with you, the reason may be due to specific nutritional deficiencies that are blocking your ability to burn fat and sugars.

Many people trying to lose weight experience extreme difficulty because of alterations in their biochemistry. There are three crucial reasons for this. One is that obese people consume calorie-rich, nutrient-poor foods. For example, processed foods, such as potato chips, are high in carbohydrates, trans fats, and salt, and they are essentially devoid of vitamins and minerals. A McDonald's Big Mac (without cheese) contains 576 calories. More than 50 percent of those calories come from fat. Therefore, eating habits of obese people often result in increased risk of diabetes and coronary artery disease at a young age.

In essence, Ronald McDonald is not a symbol of innocence; he is a symbol of obesity, heart disease, cancer, and premature death. These foods lack minerals such as chromium, vanadium, and magnesium, which are required for a healthy body and for burning fat. Obese people are actually starving themselves. This seemingly paradoxical statement reflects the inherent contradiction in trying to lose weight. Amidst a cornucopia of plenty—fruits, vegetables, lean protein sources—their body is telling them they're starving.

Another reason obese people struggle to lose weight is because they are usually depressed and anxious, and to compensate they consume more carbohydrate-rich foods to elevate their mood. And finally, because of nutrient depletions, their bodies think they are starving and send signals to the brain to eat more food. Additionally, the stress they're under from the nutrient depletions and their emotional state stimulates the secretion of cortisol in the adrenal glands. Cortisol acts to increase sugar in the bloodstream, and when there is an excess of sugar, the body turns it into fat.

This situation is what the authors call *the fat trap*. Unfortunately, our society views obesity as a fault with a person's willpower. That oversimplification is not only unrealistic, it's cruel. Sugar causes a release of serotonin in the brain, which elevates mood.[57] So people who are depressed reach for sugar to comfort themselves, which is why sweets and high-carbohydrate foods are often considered comfort foods. This is a vicious cycle: as people become more obese and depressed, they reach for more sweets in a completely futile attempt to lift themselves out of their depression.

This trap is actually two traps. One is the hormonal imbalances, and the other is the difficulty people have with sticking to healthy regimens. This is not your fault, but rather a combination of societal pressures and biochemical abnormalities. Additionally, most people never developed the tools to adequately address these traps and overcome them. This is the focus of the next section of this book, in which you will discover ways to make goals and achieve them.

Chapter 6:
Establish Your Baseline—
the MetaCT™ Test

Before diving into major life changes, it's important to know what those changes entail, and to set realistic goals. The most sustainable changes in life are those that are made gradually, in baby steps, instead of discarding the past and throwing yourself into radical change.

Most books and physicians try to help people using a shotgun approach to therapy. Some people benefit from generic diet and lifestyle recommendations. But the true revolution in health comes only with programs tailored to your specific needs. It's not that doctors don't want to provide the best recommendations possible; it's just that they're not aware of the knowledge that's available to them and to you.

The most objective way to assess what you'll need is to take test panels developed by the authors. To begin with, the MetaCT™ 400 is the most sophisticated test that medicine and nutritional biochemistry has ever seen. This is the test you need when all else has failed, and you've seen every doctor who gives you just another prescription and diagnosis that doesn't actually identify or correct the underlying problems.

The basic premises behind this testing are simple. Health and disease are biochemical in nature. If someone wasn't sick before and he is sick now, something's changed in his biochemistry. By identifying the underlying biochemical abnormalities, they can be corrected using targeted nutrient therapies to promote health and correct the underlying causes of disease. The MetaCT tests are so sophisticated that they've been called "metabolic CT scans." There are many testing options available. The most comprehensive test, the MetaCT 400, requires eight vials of blood, one vial of urine, and a stool sample, and reports more than 450 variables of biochemical function (table 6.1). Each of the sections of the MetaCT 400 test can be broken down and ordered as individual tests.

Table 6.1. Variables Reported on the MetaCT 400 Test	
Complete Blood Count with Differential	White Blood Cells (WBC), Red Blood Cells (RBC), Hemoglobin, Hematocrit, Mean Corpuscular Volume (MCV), Mean Corpuscular Hemoglobin (MCH), Mean Corpuscular Hemoglobin Content (MCHC), Red Cell Distribution Width (RDW), Platelets, Neutrophils, Lymphocytes, Mid Cells
Serum Chemistries	Fasting Blood Glucose, Urea Nitrogen (BUN), Creatinine, Total Protein, Albumin, Total Bilirubin, Calcium, Sodium, Potassium, Chloride, Carbon Dioxide, Carbon Dioxide, Alkaline Phosphatase, SGOT (AST), SGPT (ALT)
Vitamins	Coenzyme Q10, 25-Hydroxyvitamin D, Alpha-Tocopherol, Gamma-Tocopherol, Vitamin A, Beta-Carotene
Intracellular Essential Minerals	Calcium, Chromium, Copper, Magnesium, Manganese, Potassium, Selenium, Zinc
Toxic Metals	Aluminum, Arsenic, Cadmium, Lead, Mercury
Iron Panel	Serum Iron, Iron Binding Capacity, % Saturation, Serum Ferritin
Lipid Panel	Total Cholesterol, Triglycerides, HDL Cholesterol, LDL Cholesterol, Cholesterol-to-HDL Ratio, Lipoprotein(a)
Thyroid Panel	Thyroid Stimulating Hormone (TSH), Total T3, Free T4

Table 6.1. Variables Reported on the MetaCT 400 Test	
Gastrointestinal Microbiology Profile	<u>Bacteria infections</u>: *Helicobacter Pylori* (*H. pylori*), *Clostridium difficile.*, *E. coli*, *Campylobacter* spp., *Aeromonas* spp. and others <u>Fungal infections</u> (e.g., *Candida* sp.) <u>Parasitic infections</u> (e.g., *Giardia lamblia*, *Cryptosporidia* spp.) <u>Healthy gut bacteria</u>: *Bacteroides* sp., *Clostridia* sp., *Prevotella* sp., *Fusobacteria* sp., *Streptomyces* sp., *Mycoplasma* sp., *Lactobacillus* sp., *Bifidobacter* sp.
Amino Acids	<u>Essential Amino Acids (EAA)</u>: Arginine, Histidine, Isoleucine, Leucine, Lysine, Methionine, Phenylalanine, Threonine, Tryptophan, Valine <u>EAA Derivatives: Neuroendocrine Metabolism</u>: Gamma-Aminobutyric Acid, Glycine, Serine, Taurine, Tyrosine <u>EAA Derivatives: Ammonia/Energy Metabolism</u>: Alpha-Aminoadipic Acid, Asparagine, Aspartic Acid, Citrulline, Glutamic Acid, Glutamine, Ornithine <u>Sulfur Metabolism</u>: Cystine, Cytathionine, Homcysteine <u>Additional Metabolites</u>: Alpha-Amino-N-Butyric Acid, Alanine, Anserine, Beta-Alanine, Beta-Aminoisobutyric Acid, Carnosine, Ethanolamine, Homocysteine, Hydroxylysine, Hydroxyproline, 1-Methylhistidine, 3-Methylhistidine, Phosphoethanolamine, Phosphoserine, Proline, Sarcosine
Markers of Free Radical Damage	Lipid peroxides, 8-Hydroxy-2'deoxyguanosine, p-Hydroxyphenyllactate (HPLA)
Markers of Inflammation	Ferritin, Fibrinogen, High Sensitivity C-Reactive Protein (hsCRP), Quinolinate

Table 6.1. Variables Reported on the MetaCT 400 Test	
Hormones and Neurotransmitter Markers	Insulin, Testosterone, Sex Hormone Binding Globulin (SHBG), Free Androgen Index (calc.), Vanilmandelate, Homovanillate, 5-Hydroxyindoleacetate, Kynurenate
Fatty Acid Profile	Polyunsaturated Omega-3: Alpha-Linolenic Acid (ALA), Eicosapentaenoic Acid (EPA), Dosapentaenoic Acid, Docosahexaenoic Acid (DHA) Polyunsaturated Omega-6: Linoleic Acid, Gamma Linolenic Acid (GLA), Eicosadienoic Acid, Dihomogamma Linolenic Acid (DGLA), Arachidonic Acid (AA), Docosadienoic Acid, Docosatetraenoic Acid Polyunsaturated Omega-9: Mead Acid Monounsaturated: Myristoleic Acid, Palmitoleic Acid, Vaccenic Acid, Oleic Acid, 11-Eicosaenoic Acid, Erucic Acid, Nervonic Acid Saturated: Capric Acid, Lauric Acid, Myristic Acid, Palmitic Acid, Stearic Acid, Arachidic Acid, Behenic Acid, Lignoceric Acid, Hexacosanoic Acid Odd Chain: Pentadecanoic Acid, Heptadecanoic Acid, Nonadecanoic Acid, Heneicosanoic Acid Trans Fatty Acids: Palmitelaidic Acid, Total C:18 Trans Ratios (Calculated): LA/DGLA, EPA/DGLA, AA/EPA, Triene/Tetraene

Table 6.1. Variables Reported on the MetaCT 400 Test	
Urinary Organic Acids	<u>Fatty Acid Metabolism</u>: Adipate, Suberate, Ethylmalonate <u>Carbohydrate Metabolism</u>: Pyruvate, Lactate, Beta-Hydroxybutyrate <u>Energy Production (Citric Acid Cycle)</u>: Citrate, cis-Aconitate, Isocitrate, Alpha-Ketoglutarate, Succinate, Fumarate, Malate, Hydroxymethylglutarate <u>B-Complex Vitamin Markers</u>: Alpha-Ketoisovalerate, Alpha-Ketoisocaproate, Alpha-Keto-Beta-Methylvalarate, Xanthurenate, Beta-Hydroxyisovalerate <u>Methylation Cofactor Markers</u>: Methylmalonate, Formiminoglutamate <u>Detoxification Indicators</u>: 2-Methylhippurate, Orotate, Glucarate, Alpha-Hydroxybutyrate, Pyroglutamate, Sulfate
IgG 90-Food Allergy Panel	Almond, Apple, Apricot, Asparagus, Aspergillus mold, Avocado, Banana, Barley, String bean, Beef, Black pepper, Blueberry, Broccoli, Cabbage, Cantaloupe, Carrot, Casein, Cashew, Cauliflower, Celery, Chicken, Chocolate, Cinnamon, Clam, Coconut, Codfish, Coffee, Corn, Crab, Cranberry, Cucumber, Egg white, Egg yolk, Flounder, Garlic, Ginger, Grape, Grapefruit, Halibut, Honeydew, Lamb, Lemon, Lentil, Lettuce, Lima bean, Lobster, Mackerel, Malt, Milk, Mushroom, Mustard greens, Navy bean, Oat, Olive, Onion, Orange, Oyster, Green pea, Peach, Peanut, Pear, Pecan, Green pepper, Pineapple, Pinto bean, Pistachio, Pork, Potato, Rice, Rye, Salmon, Sesame, Shrimp, Soybean, Spinach, Strawberry, Sunflower, Sweet potato, Tea, Tomato, Trout, Tuna, Turkey, Vanilla, Watermelon, Walnut, Wheat, Baker's yeast, Brewer's yeast, Zucchini **Optional Additional Test:** Celiac Panel

The authors do not expect you to understand every variable that's been tested. It would be like asking you to understand the mathematics behind Newton's Law of Relativity. However, like his Law of Relativity, the authors want to present the baseline, proprietary tests they developed to give you, the reader, an idea of how thorough your body can be evaluated from head to toe without your having to go to a physician. Biochemical testing forms the basis for creating targeted nutrient plans that restore biochemical function to improve your health. This approach is so unique that the combinations of nutrients in clinically relevant dosages needed to produce results simply didn't exist. The authors were forced to create their own line of nutraceuticals specifically formulated to correct the abnormalities detected on the tests.

You should be aware that Drs. Neustadt and Pieczenik did not invent this technology, nor would they dare take credit for it. Rather, they worked with a team of biochemists in Atlanta, Georgia, who have been working on creating these tests over the past twenty years. Portions of this panel are available to other physicians; however, most physicians are not intellectually equipped to understand the underlying biochemical complexities, or how to appropriately interpret the results and implement them with their patients. The authors are in no way meaning to imply that other physicians are stupid. They just simply were never taught or exposed to the biochemistry of the body—and how nutritional biochemistry relates to signs and symptoms.

Biochemistry is a complex web of interactions involving the interplay between genetics, diet, and lifestyle. One of the earliest writings to discuss biochemical individuality was in 1902. In that year, Archibald E. Garrod, MD, a clinician in London, England, published a paper in the journal *Lancet*, detailing observations on patients with alkaptonuria. This inherited metabolic disorder causes urine to turn black when exposed to air. An accumulation of dark pigment in cartilage and skin, called ochronosis, also occurs. People with alkaptonuria typically develop arthritis in adulthood, particularly in the spine and large joints.

Dr. Garrod reported, "There are good reasons for thinking that alkaptonuria is not the manifestation of a disease but is rather the nature of an alternative course of metabolism ... If it be a correct inference from the available facts that the individuals of a species do not conform to an absolutely rigid standard of metabolism but differ slightly in their chemistry as they do in their structure, it is no more surprising that they should occasionally exhibit conspicuous deviations from the specific type of metabolism than that we should meet with such wide departures from the structural uniformity of the species as the presence of supernumerary digits or transposition of the viscera."[58] This astute observer was able to extrapolate subtle changes in biochemical function to anatomical variations.

It was not until 1956 that Roger Williams, PhD, a pioneer in nutrition who is often credited with popularizing the term *biochemical individuality*, wrote the book *Biochemical Individuality: The Basis for the Genotrophic Concept.*[59] Williams believed that people have different requirements for nutrients, and some may need much higher amounts of nutrients for their unique biochemistry to function properly. He wrote, "Individuality in nutritional needs is the basis for the genetotrophic approach and for the belief that nutrition applied with due concern for individual genetic variations, which may be large, offers the solution to many baffling health problems."

Dr. Williams had based his assertions on anatomical and physiological variations among people, and it would not be until the latter years of this last century that researchers such as Bruce Ames, PhD, a UC Berkeley biochemist, would explain the biochemical bases for these assertions. Dr. Ames applied the concept of Dr. Williams's work to studying gene-nutrient interactions. His research showed that variations in genes producing the same enzyme for a biochemical reaction commonly decrease an enzyme's binding affinity (its ability to use its cofactors). [60-63] The result is an accumulation of the reactants and decreased amounts of products, which can be corrected by providing higher amounts of the cofactors. [60-63]

Phenylketonuria (PKU) provides an excellent illustration of this concept. PKU is an autosomal recessive disorder resulting from phenylalanine hydroxylase (PAH) deficiency. [64] PAH catalyzes the reaction of phenylalanine (Phe) to tyrosine (Tyr). Decreased PAH activity results in hyperphenylalanemia, a neurotoxin that causes mental retardation. More than five hundred mutations in genes coding for PAH have been determined, resulting in PAH activity ranging from severe inhibition with PAH as low as 5 percent of normal to mild PKU with near-normal PAH function. [65] More than half of children with PKU have one of the milder phenotypes. [66]

This disorder is screened for at birth and has an incidence of one in ten thousand. Phe is found in all protein foods, and neonates diagnosed with this condition are placed on a phenylalanine-restricted diet and supplemented with Tyr, vitamins, minerals and other amino acids. While effective, maintaining this severely limited diet is quite difficult in school-age children, leads to socially awkward situations in adults, and is complicated in pregnant women.

Since 1999, several clinical trials have reported positive results in decreasing serum Phe in people with PAH deficiencies by administering pharmacological doses of tetrahydrobiopterin (BH_4), a PAH cofactor. In one small study involving five children, serum Phe concentrations declined in four of five of them, with a loading dose of 10 mg BH_4 per kilogram of body weight.[67]

A larger study conducted in 2002 stratified thirty-eight children into three groups: mild hyperphenylalinemia (pretreatment plasma phenylalanine less than 600 µmol/L), mild PKU (pretreatment plasma phenylalanine 600–1200 µmol/L) and classic or severe PKU (pretreatment plasma phenylalanine greater than 1200 µmol/L). Participants were fed a meal containing 100 mg Phe per kilogram body weight loading dose, followed one hour later with 20 mg BH_4 per kilogram body weight. Blood Phe levels were determined at baseline, before BH_4, and at four, eight, and fifteen hours after BH_4. A child whose Phe level decreased by more than 30 percent after BH_4 compared to after the Phe loading test was considered responsive to therapy. All children classified as having mild phenylalanemia and 17 of the 21 children (87 percent) responded to BH_4 treatment. Within responders, the amount of Phe decrease ranged from 37 to 92 percent. Infants and children with this disorder should now also be tested for their responsiveness to BH_4 therapy, as it may allow many of them to consume a less restrictive diet, and some to even cease the therapeutic diet altogether. What this study showed is that even in severe genetic conditions, there may be some enzyme activity that can be stimulated with pharmacologic dosages of nutrients, and that diseases once viewed as incurable may in fact be ameliorated with nutrients.

The reason we insist on explaining these concepts to you in such detail is because the authors respect their readers. The intention is to impart to you relevant information so you can understand the scientific basis underlying this revolutionary approach to health, and why it's important for you to accept it as part of your lifestyle. The authors are not insisting on a leap of faith, as many authors of other self-help books do. They are only asking you to look at it—not necessarily memorize it—so that you understand that there is a logical progression of function, from the smallest biochemical element of the cell to how you feel and how your body as a whole reacts.

It is physically impossible for the body to function optimally if its biochemistry is dysfunctional. Again, this is not new information. As far back as the 1950s, researchers identified essential amino acids and discovered that low levels of any one of them (e.g., phenylalanine, leucine, isoleucine, valine, tryptophan, etc.) caused a "failure in appetite, a sensation of extreme fatigue, and an increase in nervous irritability."[68-71] Pathways affecting mood and energy can be tested using a combination of urinary organic acids, plasma amino acids, and intracellular minerals.

Food Intolerances (Allergies)

We want to explain why these tests are so important. To do so, they will discuss the most basic test—food allergies. Symptoms of food allergies are as diverse as fatigue; anemia; joint pain; depression; loss of balance; malnutrition; skin irritations such as rashes, hives, and eczema; gastrointestinal symptoms such as nausea, gas and bloating, diarrhea, constipation, and vomiting; sneezing; runny nose; shortness of breath; recurrent ear infections in children; and brain fog (decreased ability to process information). And this is by no means an exhaustive list. Food allergies are associated with more than one hundred medical conditions and one hundred different symptoms.

People will react to foods that they crave, such as milk and eggs, which can be detected through a special blood test. The blood test most used by the authors to detect food allergies evaluates the IgG immunoglobulin. An immunoglobulin is a protein produced by the immune system to attack things the immune system senses as "foreign" and dangerous to the body. There are four classes of immunoglobulins: IgA, IgM, IgE, and IgG. The IgG blood test is called an *IgG food intolerance test*, and people with rheumatoid arthritis, eczema, and other conditions have been shown to have elevated IgG antibodies to foods.[40, 41] Most doctors only test for IgE-mediated allergies, which are also called "immediate hypersensitivity reactions." An IgE-mediated immune response is responsible for the life-threatening reaction some people have to bee stings or peanuts. IgG, on the other hand, is a delayed-type hypersensitivity reaction that, as the name implies, is not immediately apparent.[42] People who test negative on an IgE test can be positive on an IgG test.[43]

IgG reactions may take hours or days to appear, and symptoms can include postnasal drip, gas and bloating, difficulty losing weight, joint aches, eczema, fatigue, and others. Food intolerances can cause these diverse symptoms for various reasons. Similar to intestinal bacterial and fungal infections, the immune system activation caused by food intolerances can cause postnasal drip. Gas and bloating are a result of incomplete digestion of food and the resultant fermentation of these food particles by bacteria in the intestines. Difficulty losing weight may result from an increased cortisol response by the body due to the continual stress placed on the immune system. When cortisol is chronically elevated, it causes an accumulation of abdominal fat.

The explanation for eczema and joint pain is a little more complicated. When the immune system in the intestines is activated, the antibody-antigen complexes enter the bloodstream. An antibody is the protein produced by the immune system, such as IgG, and an antigen is the molecule against which the immune system is reacting, such as a protein in milk. These antibody-antigen complexes travel from the intestines to the liver, where they are broken down for elimination by the body. This process is like a conveyor belt whereby the antibody-antigen complexes are delivered to the liver for processing, but the amount of complexes delivered to the liver over time can overwhelm the liver's ability to detoxify them. When this occurs, the complexes pass through the liver and enter the systemic circulation. Like bits of sand in a river, these complexes can settle out of the bloodstream, where the flow of blood slows down. This occurs in the skin and joints. When these complexes are deposited in skin and joints, they act as irritants that can create local immune system activation and produce such symptoms as joint pain and eczema. Frequently, the joint pain will be migratory.

Urinary Organic Acids

When you go to a doctor's office and they take a routine urinalysis, the physician is looking for blood, protein, sugar, bilirubin (breakdown product of red blood cells), leukocyte esterase (an enzyme produced by some bacteria that cause urinary tract infections), nitrites, and ketones (produced by people with uncontrolled diabetes). These screen for diabetes, urinary tract infections, kidney damage, and kidney stones.

In contrast, our urinary organic acids test evaluates twenty-seven different variables. It evaluates the following range of functions: your ability to produce cellular energy through burning fat and sugars (carbohydrates); whether you're functionally deficient in any of the B vitamins (B1, B2, B3, B5, B6, biotin, B12, and folic acid), which are involved in each of the tens of thousands of biochemical reactions in the body; and if your liver detoxification pathways are impaired. This analysis at the biochemical level is the most fundamental type of evaluation possible. It literally provides data that may determine the underlying causes of fatigue, inability to lose weight, depression, brain fog, decreased exercise tolerance, insulin resistance, and more.

Here's the crucial concept that you, the reader, should understand. Our tests allows skilled clinicians to delineate the body functions and make diagnoses that would otherwise not be possible, even with a PET scan, MRI, CT scan, and all the conventional tests available. It's not uncommon for people to spend tens of thousands of dollars on conventional testing and treatments without receiving any benefit.

Gastrointestinal Microbial Ecology Profile

Normally when you go into your physician you get a routine workup. If you're over fifty years old, you may get a test called a *guiac test*. The test is a simple way to determine if you have blood in your stool, which may indicate colon cancer. If they suspect a parasitic infection, usually if you go in to the doctor complaining of gas, bloating, and diarrhea after having traveled to a third world country, they order an *ova & parasite (O&P) x 3*. In an O&Px3 test, you provide samples of your stool, which are evaluated under a microscope by a parasitologist who is literally looking for small parasite eggs or the parasites themselves. To detect a parasite, the parasitologist must rely not just on his or her skills, but also on luck. The parasitologist must be lucky enough to have a stool sample that by chance had a large enough parasite or parasite egg in it to be seen through a microscope. They do not look at every square centimeter of the stool, but take samples from the stool to look at. They therefore must also be lucky that the random sample they took had something in it. This test is highly unreliable.

Table 6.2. Symptoms of parasite infections
All skin problems
Anal itching (especially at night)
Any menstrual complaint
Arthritic pain
Bed-wetting
Burning in the stomach
Chronic candida
Chronic fatigue
Chronic sinus or ear infections
Chronic viral syndromes
Constipation
Crawling feeling under the skin
Cysts and fibroids
Depression
Diarrhea
Digestive problems
Drooling while sleeping
Eating more and still being hungry
Floaters
Forgetfulness
Gas and bloating
Grinding teeth
Heart pain
Hemorrhoids
Inability to gain or lose weight
Irritable bowel syndrome
Itchy ears or nose
Liver/gallbladder trouble
Mucous in stools
Numb hands
Pain in the back (thighs or shoulders)

Table 6.2. Symptoms of parasite infections
Pain in the navel
Prostate problems
Sexual dysfunction in men
Urinary tract infections
Water retention (mostly from tapeworms)
Yeast infections

The authors' tests are based on a new paradigm in medicine—nutritional biochemistry—and new technology that is more sensitive and specific than older, outdated tests. The stool sample in this next generation of tests is automated and evaluates DNA fragments in the stool. This eliminates the role of luck in the process. Instead, the stool sample is run through a sophisticated machine. The stool sample does not need to have an intact parasite or egg in it. Instead, all that's needed are five cells from the parasite or egg to be detected.

Additionally, from this one stool sample, the tests can detect *H. pylori* infection in the stomach, bacterial and yeast infections in the intestines, and whether your intestines are low in healthy bacteria. *H. pylori* is a bacterium that colonizes in the stomach and is considered a Type I carcinogen, meaning that it causes cancer in humans. Most physicians will not test for any of these other infections, even though the symptoms significantly overlap with those of a parasite infection.

Parasitic diagnoses are rare because most physicians are not trained in parasitology. It's a rare medical school that exposes students to a six- or eight-week course in parasitology. Most standard medical evaluations do not include a parasite test, and even when they do, it's an extremely insensitive test. Why might it be important to test for parasites? Because the symptoms mimic many other diseases. For a list of symptoms that can be caused by parasites, see table 6.2.

Chapter 7:
Create and Implement Your Program

Based on your health history, family history, present condition, and test results, a customized health program is created for you. In all the years of helping people this way, Dr. Neustadt has never created two plans that are exactly alike because no two people or their biochemistries are exactly alike. The promise of individualized, personalized medicine is here.

But there are some important things you can start doing today to help yourself. First, make sure you're protecting yourself from environmental toxins. Drink filtered water, buy organic foods, and do not eat fish contaminated with toxic metals (e.g., shark and tuna). We understand that most everyone is on a budget and may not be able to afford to eat all organic. Therefore, we provide a list of the foods that are most contaminated and should only be eaten if they're certified organic. They call these "the dirty dozen."

The Dirty Dozen: Twelve Foods to Buy Organic

The dirty dozen are the foods most commonly and highly contaminated with pesticides and chemicals, even after washing and peeling. FDA and USDA research shows high levels of pesticide and chemical contamination in these common foods. The research used to compile this list is from extensive independent tests run by the FDA and the USDA from more than one hundred thousand samples of food. The chemical pesticides detected in these studies are known to cause cancer, birth defects, nervous system and brain damage, and developmental problems in children. In other words, *eat organic*.

Many people want to eat organically grown and certified food, but find it too expensive to eat all organic. To help readers prioritize which foods they should purchase that are certified organic, they compiled the following list.

Beef, Pork, and Poultry

The EPA reports that meat is contaminated with higher levels of pesticides than any plant food. Many chemical pesticides are fat-soluble and accumulate in the fatty tissue of animals. Animal feed that contains animal products compounds the accumulation, which is directly passed to the human consumer. Antibiotics, drugs, and hormones are a standard in animal husbandry, all of which accumulate and are passed on to consumers as well. Ocean fish carry a higher risk for heavy metals than pesticides, though many freshwater fish are exposed to high levels of pesticides from contaminated water.

Milk, Cheese, and Butter

For reasons similar to those for meat, the fat in dairy products poses a high risk for contamination by pesticides. Animals concentrate pesticides and chemicals in their milk and meat. Growth hormones and antibiotics are also serious concerns and are invariably found in commercial milk, cheese, and butter.

Strawberries, Raspberries, and Cherries

In America, strawberries are the crop most heavily dosed with pesticides in America. On average, three hundred pounds of pesticides are applied to every acre of strawberries (compared to an average of twenty-five pounds per acre for other foods). Thirty-six different pesticides are commonly used on strawberries, and 90 percent of strawberries tested register pesticide contamination above safe levels. Raspberries trump strawberries, with the application of thirty-nine chemicals: 58 percent of raspberries tested registered positive for contamination. Cherries are equally concerning, with twenty-five pesticides and 91 percent contamination.

Apples and Pears

With thirty-six different chemicals detected in FDA testing, half of which are neurotoxins (meaning they cause brain damage), apples are almost as contaminated as strawberries. In fact, 91 percent of apples tested positive for pesticide residue. Peeling nonorganic apples reduces but does not eliminate the danger of ingesting these chemicals. Pears rank hazardously near apples, with thirty-five pesticides and 94 percent contamination.

Tomatoes

It's standard practice for more than thirty pesticides to be sprayed on conventionally grown tomatoes. The thin skin does not stop chemicals from infiltrating the whole tomato, so peeling won't help you here.

Potatoes

Potatoes are one of the most popular vegetables, but they also rank among the most contaminated with pesticides and fungicides. Twenty-nine pesticides are commonly used, and 79 percent of potatoes tested exceed safe levels of multiple pesticides.

Spinach and Other Greens

The FDA found spinach to be the vegetable most frequently contaminated with the most potent pesticides used on food. Of the conventionally grown spinach that was tested, 83 percent was contaminated with dangerous levels of at least some of the thirty-six chemical pesticides commonly used to grow it.

Coffee

Most coffee is grown in countries where there are little to no standards regulating the use of chemicals and pesticides on food. The United States produces and exports millions of tons of pesticides, some of which are so dangerous that they are illegal to use on American farmland. Foreign countries import these chemicals to cultivate food that is sold back to the United States. Coffee is an unfortunate culprit in this vicious cycle of agriculture. Purchasing fair trade coffee provides insurance that the premium price paid for this treasured beverage supports farms and workers with more equanimity and reward.

Peaches and Nectarines

Forty-five different pesticides are regularly applied to succulent, delicious peaches and nectarines in conventional orchards. The thin skin does not protect the fruit from the dangers of these poisons. Of those tested for pesticide residue, 97 percent of nectarines and 95 percent of peaches show contamination from multiple chemicals.

Grapes

Because grapes are a delicate fruit, they are sprayed multiple times during different stages of growth. The thin skin does not offer much protection from the thirty-five different pesticides used as a standard in conventional vineyards. Imported grapes are even more heavily treated than grapes grown in the United States. Several of the most poisonous pesticides banned in the United States are still used on grapes grown abroad. The portion of grapes testing positive for pesticide contamination is 86 percent, with samples from Chile showing the highest concentration of the most poisonous chemicals.

Celery

Conventionally grown celery is subjected to at least twenty-nine different chemicals, which cannot be washed off because celery does not have any protective skin. Of celery tested, 94 percent had pesticide residues in violation of safe levels.

Red and Green Bell Peppers

Bell Peppers are one of the most heavily sprayed foods, with standard use of thirty-nine pesticides. In fact, 68 percent of bell peppers tested had high levels of chemical pesticide residues. The thin skin of the pepper does not offer much protection from spraying, and it is often waxed with harmful substances.

Exercise and Breathe

It's important to exercise and increase your respiration rate. Oxygen is often overlooked as an essential nutrient. Every tissue is bathed in oxygen, but most people breathe shallowly and do not get enough physical activity. You may want to begin by having a trainer evaluate you and put you on a physical fitness program that's safe and effective for you. If you are at an elevated risk for heart or respiratory diseases, then you need to speak with your doctor before exercising. Some of these risk factors include having had a previous heart attack, being overweight, being over the age of fifty, having been diagnosed with coronary artery disease, and having high blood pressure or diabetes.

Chapter 8:
Cases in Nutritional Biochemistry

All cases presented here were interpreted only by Dr. Neustadt.

Age-Related Degeneration (ARD)

Age-related degeneration (ARD) is a term created by Drs. Neustadt and Pieczenik to describe a constellation of symptoms that tend to appear in the elderly. These symptoms may include weakness, fatigue, depression, insomnia, abdominal gas and bloating, diarrhea, brain fog (difficulty processing information), and recurrent infections, such as urinary tract infections (UTI) and/or upper respiratory infections (URI).

In these people, conventional medical testing usually does not show any abnormalities, and all treatments merely suppress symptoms without addressing the underlying causes. It is well documented that as we age, our risk for nutritional deficiencies increases,[72] and the underlying causes for these symptoms include deficiencies in amino acid, vitamins, minerals, and fatty acids, as well as food allergies and intestinal dysbiosis (overgrowth of bacteria and/or yeast). Biochemical testing can provide the information needed to create a Targeted Nutritional Program™ that can help restore health.

Case: Muscle Wasting / Fatigue / Weakness / Muscle Pain / Gas and Bloating / Diarrhea

A sixty-nine-year-old woman went to see Dr. Neustadt at the Montana Integrative Medicine clinic complaining of extreme fatigue, weakness, muscle pain, severe gas and bloating each time she ate, and a five-year history of loose stools. When she walked less than one block, she experienced painful burning in her muscles. At intake, she could only walk half a block and ride for one minute on a stationery bicycle. Additionally, she was unable to stand up from a seated position on the floor without assistance. She was losing strength and balance, which put her at a high risk for falling and hip fractures.

She had been evaluated by gastroenterologists, internists, gynecologists, and urologists at major medical centers around the country. None of them found any abnormalities. Biochemical testing revealed deficiencies in seven out of ten amino acids, low vitamins and minerals required for mitochondrial function, an intestinal bacterial infection, and multiple food allergies.

Low amino acids			
Arginine	50	L	63
Histidine	65	L	67
Isoleucine	45	L	47
Leucine	85	L	87
Lysine	152		135
Methionine	16	L	18
Phenylalanine	53		50
Threonine	72	L	90
Tryptophan	43		42
Valine	168		167
Glycine	154	L	186
Serine	56	L	77

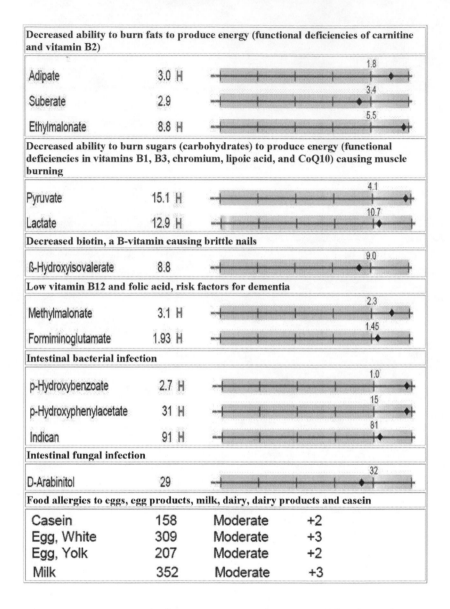

Decreased ability to burn fats to produce energy (functional deficiencies of carnitine and vitamin B2)			
Adipate	3.0 H		1.8
Suberate	2.9		3.4
Ethylmalonate	8.8 H		5.5
Decreased ability to burn sugars (carbohydrates) to produce energy (functional deficiencies in vitamins B1, B3, chromium, lipoic acid, and CoQ10) causing muscle burning			
Pyruvate	15.1 H		4.1
Lactate	12.9 H		10.7
Decreased biotin, a B-vitamin causing brittle nails			
ß-Hydroxyisovalerate	8.8		9.0
Low vitamin B12 and folic acid, risk factors for dementia			
Methylmalonate	3.1 H		2.3
Formiminoglutamate	1.93 H		1.45
Intestinal bacterial infection			
p-Hydroxybenzoate	2.7 H		1.0
p-Hydroxyphenylacetate	31 H		15
Indican	91 H		81
Intestinal fungal infection			
D-Arabinitol	29		32
Food allergies to eggs, egg products, milk, dairy, dairy products and casein			
Casein	158	Moderate	+2
Egg, White	309	Moderate	+3
Egg, Yolk	207	Moderate	+2
Milk	352	Moderate	+3

Her treatment consisted of instructions to eliminate all food intolerances, take antibacterial plant extracts for the intestinal infection, high doses of B-complex vitamins with extra vitamin B12, a customized amino acid powder, a high-quality multivitamin and mineral supplement, and physical therapy. Two months later, she could walk pain free for twenty minutes twice daily and ride for ten minutes on an exercise bike. She no longer suffered from diarrhea, and her gas and bloating had also improved. Additionally, she was able to stand up from a seated position without assistance.

Case 2: Weight loss / Decreased Strength / Gas and Bloating / Postnasal Drip

An eighty-one-year-old man was complaining of progressive weight loss, which had been occurring for the past ten years, decreased strength, flatulence, and postnasal drip. He had been losing weight for twelve years, had been worked up by numerous physicians without any relief, and had dropped to a low of 139 pounds, which bordered on undernutrition.

Multiple, severe amino acid deficiencies. In such cases the body will break down muscle protein, so repleting amino acids is crucial to correcting this condition.

Arginine	51	50 - 160	
Histidine	65 L	70 - 140	
Isoleucine	43 L	50 - 160	
Leucine	76 L	90 - 200	
Lysine	134 L	150 - 300	
Methionine	24 L	25 - 50	
Phenylalanine	45	45 - 140	
Threonine	82 L	100 - 250	
Tryptophan	35	35 - 65	
Valine	135 L	170 - 420	
Glycine	212 L	225 - 450	
Serine	74 L	90 - 210	
Taurine	43 L	50 - 250	
Tyrosine	41 L	50 - 120	

Low and low-normal essential minerals

Chromium	0.29	
Copper	0.53	
Magnesium	48	
Manganese	0.23 L	
Potassium	1,759	
Selenium	0.14	
Vanadium	0.11	
Zinc	6.4	

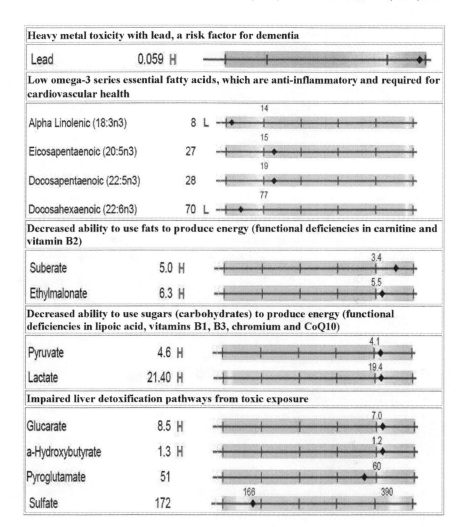

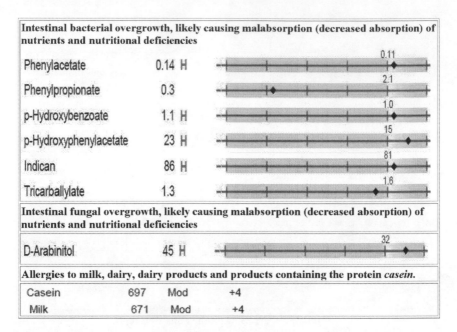

Intestinal bacterial overgrowth, likely causing malabsorption (decreased absorption) of nutrients and nutritional deficiencies		
Phenylacetate	0.14 H	0.11
Phenylpropionate	0.3	2.1
p-Hydroxybenzoate	1.1 H	1.0
p-Hydroxyphenylacetate	23 H	15
Indican	86 H	81
Tricarballylate	1.3	1.6

Intestinal fungal overgrowth, likely causing malabsorption (decreased absorption) of nutrients and nutritional deficiencies		
D-Arabinitol	45 H	32

Allergies to milk, dairy, dairy products and products containing the protein *casein*.			
Casein	697	Mod	+4
Milk	671	Mod	+4

He was placed on a Targeted Nutritional Program to correct his nutritional deficiencies, which included a customized amino acid powder and specific blends of vitamins, minerals, and fatty acids. His intestinal infections were treated using antibacterial and antifungal agents. He followed a gut restoration protocol to repair any damage to his intestines that the infections may have caused, and he began a series of intravenous chelation treatments under the care of Dr. Neustadt in his clinic, Montana Integrative Medicine. His postnasal drip cleared up, his strength increased, and his weight went up to 149 pounds.

Arthritis

Arthritis is a painful inflammation of the joints. There are many different types of arthritis, including rheumatoid arthritis, osteoarthritis, and psoriatic arthritis. In these conditions, specific joints are affected, which can make it difficult to open a jar, tie your shoes, and participate in sports or other enjoyable activities. Arthritis can also be migratory.

Case: Severe Joint Pain / Muscle Pain / Restless Leg Syndrome / Constipation

A forty-one-year-old man complained of severe joint and muscle pain that started three years earlier. The pain was so severe that he said it felt like his "whole body was in a pressure suit." He was unable to enjoy basic activities because of the pain. Additionally, he also suffered from insomnia, restless leg syndrome, and constipation. It would take him an hour of lying in bed to fall asleep, and his restless leg syndrome would wake him up multiple times during the night. He would only have a bowel movement every four to five days.

His MetaCT 400 test results revealed:

Amino acid deficiencies

Arginine	52	50 - 160	
Histidine	78	70 - 140	
Isoleucine	47 L	50 - 160	
Leucine	97	90 - 200	
Lysine	155	150 - 300	
Methionine	24 L	25 - 50	
Phenylalanine	44 L	45 - 140	
Threonine	152	100 - 250	
Tryptophan	28 L	35 - 65	
Valine	187	170 - 420	
Glycine	250	225 - 450	
Serine	87 L	90 - 210	
Taurine	60	50 - 250	
Tyrosine	53	50 - 120	

Mineral deficiency of manganese, which is required as an antioxidant

Manganes	32	

Deficiencies in antioxidants

Coenzyme Q10	0.54	
Vitamin A	0.50 L	
ß-Carotene	0.21 L	

Elevated 8-Hydroxy-2-deoxyguanosine, indicating free radical damage to DNA, a risk factor for cancer and other conditions

8-Hydroxy-2-deoxyguanosine	5.8 H	

Low vitamin D

25-Hydroxyvitamin D	21	

Low fatty acids (omega-3 polyunsaturated fatty acids and saturated fatty acids). Omega-3 fatty acids are anti-inflammatory.		
Alpha Linolenic (18:3n3)	7 L	14
Eicosapentaenoic (20:5n3)	4 L	15
Docosapentaenoic (22:5n3)	13 L	19
Docosahexaenoic (22:6n3)	45 L	77

Low sulfate, required for liver detoxification and for connective tissue formation		
Sulfate	125 L	166 390

Food allergies			
Casein	1,058	Severe	+5
Egg, White	1,408	Severe	+5
Egg, Yolk	1,447	Severe	+5
Milk	> 2000	Severe	+5
Peanut	1,597	Severe	+5
Pistachio	582	Mod	+4
Mustard Greens	240	Mod	+3
Spinach	151	Mod	+3

He was instructed to eliminate food allergies for eight weeks while following a gut restoration program. Specific nutrients were also recommended to him as dietary supplements to correct his underlying deficiencies. After two weeks on the program, this gentleman reported that his restless leg syndrome decreased by 80 percent, he no longer experienced any insomnia, his muscle pain and cramps decreased by 70 percent, and he no longer had any constipation. At the end of his program, after three months, he reported that he no longer suffered from any restless leg syndrome, brain fog, constipation, and muscle or joint pain. All his initial complaints had completely resolved.

Case: Migratory Arthritis / Metabolic Syndrome (Prediabetes) / Fatigue / Restlessness / Depression / Obesity

A forty-eight-year-old woman suffered for five years with migratory, polyarticular (multiple joints) joint pain throughout her body; however, the joints most affected were her knees, ankles, and hands. Her joint pain was debilitating, keeping her from her favorite pastime, riding horses. She used to raise horses, and at one time had thirty horses. She also complained of pain, fatigue, restlessness, depression, and being overweight. When she was first evaluated, her energy was between four and five (ten being best), and she reported days when her energy was zero out of ten. She slept three to four hours nightly, although she said that she would actually lie in bed for up to eight hours each night. She suffered from insomnia, with difficulty falling asleep. Her stress had been quite high, and she rated it a nine and a half out of ten (ten being worst) for the four to five years prior. She was also overweight and unable to drop the excess pounds.Her goal was to feel well enough to ride horses again.

She took the MetaCT 400 test and her results revealed:

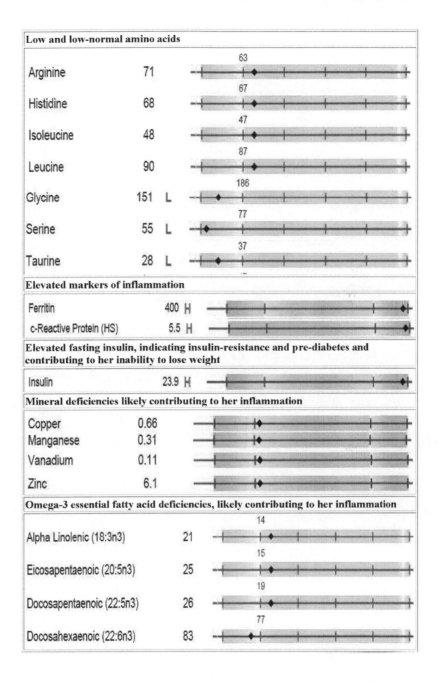

Low and low-normal amino acids		
Arginine	71	63
Histidine	68	67
Isoleucine	48	47
Leucine	90	87
Glycine	151 L	186
Serine	55 L	77
Taurine	28 L	37

Elevated markers of inflammation

Ferritin	400 H
c-Reactive Protein (HS)	5.5 H

Elevated fasting insulin, indicating insulin-resistance and pre-diabetes and contributing to her inability to lose weight

Insulin	23.9 H

Mineral deficiencies likely contributing to her inflammation

Copper	0.66
Manganese	0.31
Vanadium	0.11
Zinc	6.1

Omega-3 essential fatty acid deficiencies, likely contributing to her inflammation

Alpha Linolenic (18:3n3)	21	14
Eicosapentaenoic (20:5n3)	25	15
Docosapentaenoic (22:5n3)	26	19
Docosahexaenoic (22:6n3)	83	77

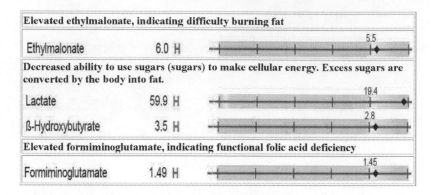

Elevated ethylmalonate, indicating difficulty burning fat		
Ethylmalonate	6.0 H	5.5
Decreased ability to use sugars (sugars) to make cellular energy. Excess sugars are converted by the body into fat.		
Lactate	59.9 H	19.4
ß-Hydroxybutyrate	3.5 H	2.8
Elevated formiminoglutamate, indicating functional folic acid deficiency		
Formiminoglutamate	1.49 H	1.45

This woman was provided dietary and exercise recommendations to help her lose weight. She was referred to a physical trainer to put her on a therapeutic exercise program. She also began taking specific dietary supplements to correct her nutritional deficiencies and improve her ability to burn her sugars and fats for energy. While on the program, her joint pain resolved, her energy increased, her food cravings for sugar decreased, her insomnia went away, and she finally began to lose weight after years of frustrations.

Asthma

Asthma is a respiratory condition characterized by decreased ability to breathe, and it is accompanied by wheezing, shortness of breath, and, in severe attacks, death. This is caused by bronchoconstriction, which means the airway (bronchi) is narrowing (constricting) so there is a decrease in oxygen flow. Asthma can occur in children and in adults. In children, food allergies are frequently present. Identifying these allergies with an IgG antibody test can be helpful, as can recommending anti-inflammatory dietary supplements to decrease inflammation in the lungs. In contrast, adult onset asthma, also called mature-onset asthma, occurs in adults who have no history of asthma. In adults, this condition is frequently caused by decreased production of epinephrine, a compound the body normally creates that, among other things, causes the lungs to dilate so people can breathe. The nutrients required to produce epinephrine include the amino acid tyrosine, vitamin B6, copper, and iron.

Case: Mature Onset Asthma / Prediabetes

This is the case of Dr. Pieczenik, the founder of NBITC. When he was sixty-two years old, he presented at Montana Integrative Medicine with a previous diagnosis of mature-onset exercise-induced asthma. This condition develops in adults and results in a decreased ability to breathe during exercise or cold weather. In his case, his lungs would constrict and his pulmonologist determined that he had a 22 percent deficit in oxygen. He was literally short of breath all the time. While his pulmonologist could not determine the cause of the dysfunction, he nonetheless wanted to treat it symptomatically with steroids. Steroids have been around for more than forty years, and Dr. Pieczenik could not believe that there had been no advances in medicine during that time. Steroids carry serious risk for side effects and do nothing to cure the patient; therefore, the gentleman decided to get a second opinion.

Having heard of Dr. Neustadt's work in nutritional biochemistry, he received a complete evaluation. His results showed that he had elevated tyrosine, low copper, a low copper-to-zinc ratio, and low epinephrine. Tyrosine flows down its pathway to form epinephrine and requires several vitamins and minerals to do so, including copper.

His MetaCT 400 test results revealed:

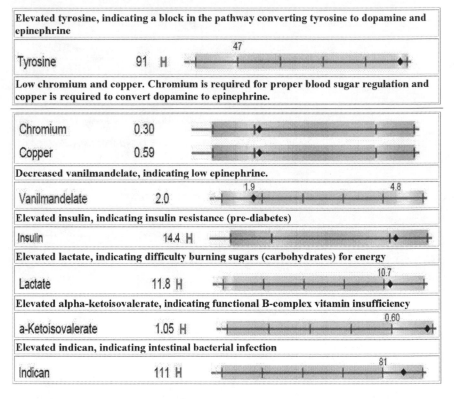

Epinephrine is a bronchodilator, and his deficiency in epinephrine was the immediate reason he developed mature onset asthma. The block in the pathway was at the step where dopamine is converted to norepinephrine, which requires copper. In turn, his deficiency in copper resulted from his chronic consumption of an over-the-counter dietary supplement containing high amounts of zinc without any copper in it. He was taking 50 mg of zinc daily because he had read somewhere that zinc may be helpful for his prostate; however, high amounts of zinc can decrease copper absorption. In effect, this patient induced a copper deficiency—and his medical condition.

By correcting his copper deficiencyall his breathing symptoms disappeared, and upon retesting several months later, his tyrosine, copper, and vanilmandelate levels had all normalized. What's important here is that the evaluation identified the underlying cause of his condition, which was treatable. His medical doctors would never even have known or understood the basic underlying functional biochemistry that led to this disorder. It was never part of their medical school education, and it still is not taught in conventional medical programs. Instead of merely providing steroids that at best may have only relieved the symptoms, the treatment here was to correct the underlying copper deficiency. Within two weeks of initiating the treatment plan to rebalance his biochemistry, the patient's mature onset asthma completely resolved. He no longer requires any steroids. Additionally, over time his insulin resistance was also corrected and he no longer had prediabetes.

Attention Deficit Hyperactivity Disorder (ADHD)

Attention Deficit Hyperactivity Disorder (ADHD) is a condition that becomes apparent in some children in the preschool and early school years. It is hard for these children to control their behavior and/or pay attention. It is estimated that between 3 and 5 percent of children have ADHD, or approximately 2 million children in the United States. This means that in a classroom of 25 to 30 children, it is likely that at least one will have ADHD.

The principal characteristics of ADHD are inattention, hyperactivity, and impulsivity. These symptoms appear early in a child's life, but can also occur in adults. Because many normal children may have these symptoms, but at a low level, or the symptoms may be caused by another disorder, it is important that the child receive a thorough examination and appropriate diagnosis by a well-qualified professional. The conventional approach to ADHD is to prescribe medications such as Adderrall, Concerta, Cylert, Dexedrine, Focalin, Metadate, and Ritalin.

Case: A mother brought her seven-year-old son to Montana Integrative Medicine for an evaluation for ADHD. He had been having troubles in school, including difficulty concentrating, angry outbursts, and disruptive behaviors. He also exhibited some of these symptoms at home, would frequently complain of stomachaches, and had previously been diagnosed with ADHD. His biochemical testing revealed severe food allergies to milk and wheat, an intestinal bacterial infection, and functional deficiencies in vitamin B6 and folic acid.

His intestinal bacterial infection was treated; he avoided milk, dairy products, and wheat; and he was prescribed dietary supplements for his deficiencies. The boy understood that his behaviors were damaging, and once the results were explained to him, he agreed to comply with the recommendations. At his follow up several weeks later, both he and his mother reported that all his symptoms had improved, and that he was no longer having any difficulties in school.

Bipolar Disorder

Bipolar disorder, also called manic-depressive illness, is a disorder characterized by dramatic, and sometimes rapid, mood swings. People may go from being overly energetic ("high") and/or irritable, to sad and hopeless, and then back again. They often have normal moods in between. Bipolar disorder can run in families, and people with a first-degree relative (e.g., mother, father, siblings) with this disorder run a seven times greater risk than people in the general population of having bipolar disorder. This disorder usually starts in late adolescence or early adulthood.

Bipolar disorder, or manic-depressive illness, has been recognized since at least the time of Hippocrates, who described such patients as "amic" and "melancholic." In 1899, Emil Kraepelin defined manic-depressive illness and noted that persons with manic-depressive illness lacked deterioration and dementia, which he associated with schizophrenia. Conventional medicine has no explanation of the underlying causes of bipolar disorder.

Case: Rapid Cycling Bipolar Disorder

A twenty-five-year-old man presented to Montana Integrative Medicine for an appointment with Dr. Neustadt. This patient was complaining of suffering from alternating severe anxiety and depression for the past seven years. Several years earlier, his sister was diagnosed with bipolar disorder, and his maternal grandfather suffered from depression and committed suicide. He had tried some natural therapies for his anxiety in the past, including kava kava, St. John's wort, yarrow root and skullcap. These were all helpful immediately afterwards, but they gave no long-term benefits. Counseling with a therapist did not help. He was prescribed Xanax to help with the anxiety until his test results came back and the underlying biochemical abnormalities could be treated.

Low essential amino acids and elevated ethanolamine, which has been associated with the onset of bipolar disorder and depression		
Arginine	58	
Histidine	64	L
Isoleucine	42	L
Leucine	86	L
Lysine	152	
Methionine	32	
Phenylalanine	46	
Threonine	134	
Tryptophan	39	
Valine	147	L
Serine	94	
Taurine	69	
Ethanolamine	10	H

Low minerals (note: magnesium and manganese are required to process and lower the amino acid ethanolamine, above)	
Chromium	0.29
Copper	0.63
Magnesium	45
Manganese	0.25

Low omega-3 series polyunsaturated fatty acids		
Alpha Linolenic (18:3n3)	9 L	14
Eicosapentaenoic (20:5n3)	11 L	15
Docosapentaenoic (22:5n3)	26	19
Docosahexaenoic (22:6n3)	31 L	77
Elevated xanthurenate, indicating functional vitamin B6 deficiency		
Xanthurenate	1.21 H	0.70
Decreased epinephrine (vanilmandelate) and serotonin (5-Hydroxyindoleacetate), associated with fatigue and depression		
Vanilmandelate	2.0	1.9 4.8
5-Hydroxyindoleacetate	1.5	1.5 5.6

The man was placed on nutraceuticals to correct his underlying biochemical abnormalities. After two weeks on the program he reported feeling "good," and that he had only had one bad day in the past two weeks, which was caused by his not eating and not taking his nutraceuticals. After six weeks on the program, the patient reported having no depression or anxiety for more than a month. He felt his mood was "stable," and his mood was not cycling. All his symptoms resolved, and after six months, he continued to have no symptoms of bipolar disorder.

Cancer

In the United States, cancer is responsible for about 25 percent of all deaths each year. In the United States, breast cancer is the most prevalent cancer in women, and the second most common cause of cancer death in women (after lung cancer). In 2007, breast cancer caused 40,910 deaths (7 percent of cancer deaths; almost 2 percent of all deaths) in the United States. Over their lifetimes, women in the States have a one in eight chance of developing invasive breast cancer, and a one in thirty-three chance of breast cancer causing their death. The number of cases has significantly increased since the 1970s, a phenomenon partly blamed on modern lifestyles in the Western world.

Surgery, radiation, and chemotherapy are frequently used alone and in combination to treat cancer. Each can be lifesaving, and each can cause severe side effects. Radiation can effectively kill cancerous tissue; however, radiation is nonspecific and will also damage non-target tissues. Specifically, radiation will damage those cells that divide most rapidly, which include those lining the intestines, leading to increased risk for gastrointestinal complaints, malabsorption, and nutritional deficiencies.

Chemotherapy, like many medications, causes depletions in specific nutrients. For example, Herceptin, used to treat breast cancer, can cause cardiotoxicity because it depletes L-carnitine and coenzyme Q10 (CoQ10). Testing someone's unique nutritional biochemical status and designing plans for her based on her needs can help speed up healing time from surgery, decrease side effects from radiation and chemotherapy, and improve overall strength, sense of well-being, and vitality. A team that contains doctors who are experts in nutritional biochemistry, conventional medical oncologists, body workers such as acupuncturists and massage therapists, and support groups provides the most comprehensive approach to fighting cancer. Nutritional treatments must be timed properly with radiation and chemotherapy to avoid potential interactions.

Case: Breast Cancer / Fatigue / Insomnia / Muscle Aches / Muscle Cramps / Severe Indigestion

A fifty-four-year-old woman presented to Montana Integrative Medicine after being diagnosed with breast cancer and undergoing a radical mastectomy, radiation, and chemotherapy. She continued to be on intravenous Herceptin treatments for the cancer. She complained of severe indigestion, fatigue, insomnia, constipation, muscle aching, and spasms. She rated her energy at four out of ten, ten being best. Her nutritional biochemical test revealed multiple severe deficiencies that explained most of her symptoms.

Severe amino acid deficiencies, suggesting damage to the intestines and malabsorption			
Arginine	44 L	50 - 160	
Histidine	62 L	70 - 140	
Isoleucine	47 L	50 - 160	
Leucine	72 L	90 - 200	
Lysine	128 L	150 - 300	
Methionine	23 L	25 - 50	
Phenylalanine	38 L	45 - 140	
Threonine	142	100 - 250	
Tryptophan	25 L	35 - 65	
Valine	158 L	170 - 420	
Tyrosine	38 L	50 - 120	
Glutamine	397 L	600 - 1,050	
Proline	102 L	130 - 400	

Low essential minerals		
Chromium	0.22 L	
Copper	0.48 L	
Magnesium	27 L	
Manganese	0.27	
Selenium	0.11 L	
Zinc	5.6 L	

Low omega-3 series polyunsaturated fatty acids, which are anti-inflammatory

Alpha Linolenic (18:3n3)	13 L	14
Eicosapentaenoic (20:5n3)	23	15
Docosapentaenoic (22:5n3)	28	19
Docosahexaenoic (22:6n3)	63 L	77

Decreased ability to burn fat for energy; functional deficiency in L-carnitine

Adipate	2.4 H	1.8
Suberate	3.4	3.4

Decreased ability to use carbohydrates for energy; functional deficiencies in vitamins B1, B3, lipoic acid and CoQ10

Pyruvate	6.8 H	4.1

Specific indicators of functional CoQ10 deficiency

Fumarate	2.71 H	0.71
Malate	4.3 H	2.3

Specific indicators for functional deficiencies in vitamins B1, B2, B3, B5, B6 and B12

a-Keto-ß-Methylvalerate	1.7 H	1.6
Xanthurenate	1.19 H	0.70
Methylmalonate	2.2	2.3

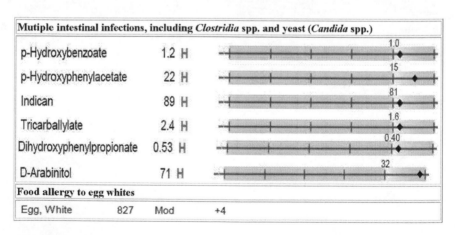

Mutiple intestinal infections, including *Clostridia* spp. and yeast (*Candida* spp.)

p-Hydroxybenzoate	1.2 H	1.0
p-Hydroxyphenylacetate	22 H	15
Indican	89 H	81
Tricarballylate	2.4 H	1.6
Dihydroxyphenylpropionate	0.53 H	0.40
D-Arabinitol	71 H	32

Food allergy to egg whites

Egg, White	827	Mod	+4

She was placed on a therapeutic program tailored specifically to her needs, which included diet and nutraceuticals. Over the next several months, her muscle cramps, indigestion, and constipation completely resolved, and her energy increased to eight out of ten (ten being best). Moreover, she described a general increase in vitality and strength.

Crohn's disease

Crohn's disease (CD), also known as regional enteritis, is a chronic, episodic, inflammatory condition of the gastrointestinal tract. CD is a type of inflammatory bowel disease (IBD). The other type is ulcerative colitis (UC). CD can affect any part of the gastrointestinal tract from mouth to anus, whereas UC primarily affects the descending colon. Symptoms of CD vary between affected individuals, with the main gastrointestinal symptoms being abdominal pain, sometimes bloody diarrhea, and weight loss. CD can also cause complications outside of the gastrointestinal tract, such as skin rashes, arthritis, and inflammation of the eye. Frequently, people with CD will undergo surgery to remove part of their intestines and will thereafter require a pouch (ileostomy) that attaches to their bowels through their abdominal wall, to collect their stool. CD patients are at extremely high risks for nutritional deficiencies.

Case: Crohn's Disease / Fatigue / Weakness / Postnasal Drip

A sixty-five-year-old woman presented to Montana Integrative Medicine with CD. She had been diagnosed forty-three years earlier, in 1964, and had undergone a hemicolectomy (partial surgical removal of her large intestine). She suffered from extreme fatigue, insomnia, weakness, and chronic postnasal drip. She reported that her energy was very low.

Her test results revealed deficiencies in branched chain amino acids (leucine, isoleucine, and valine) required to form muscle; low minerals (magnesium, copper, and vanadium); extremely low vitamin D2; elevated free radical damage to DNA, a risk factor for cancer; an intestinal fungal infection, sometimes called "intestinal candida"; and decreased ability to utilize sugars to produce energy due to functional deficiencies in B-complex vitamins and lipoic acid. Additionally, she had food allergies to milk, casein (a protein found in high concentrations in milk and dairy products, and added to many packaged foods), eggs, garlic, and mustard greens.

Amino acid deficiencies		
Isoleucine	44 L	
Leucine	75 L	
Valine	146 L	
Amino Acids		
Magnesium	30 L	
Copper	0.67	
Vanadium	0.12	
Elevated DNA free radical damage		
8-Hydroxy-2-deoxyguanosine	5.4 H	
Low vitamin D2		
25-hydroxyvitamin D	16	
Difficulty utilizing sugars for energy		
Pyruvate	4.9 H	
Lactate	18.3	19.4
Intestinal dysbiosis (overgrowth of yeast)		
D-Arabinitol	38 H	
Food allergies			
Casein	> 2000	Severe	+5
Egg, White	> 2000	Severe	+5
Egg, Yolk	366	Mod	+3
Milk	> 2000	Severe	+5
Garlic	187	Mod	+3
Mustard Greens	452	Mod	+3

She was placed on a customized program that included dietary recommendations, targeted nutrient therapies to provided highly concentrated sources of nutrients, and a protocol to eliminate the infection in her intestines. After three months on the program, she reported that her energy had doubled, saying, "I haven't felt this good in twenty-five years." Her postnasal drip had cleared up, she was sleeping better, and she felt stronger and more positive about herself and her health.

Depression

Depression is a clinical diagnosis, meaning lab tests are not used to identify depression. Symptoms vary from person to person and cause changes in thinking, feeling, behavior, and physical well-being, including difficulty concentrating and making decisions, forgetfulness, negative thoughts (e.g., pessimism, poor self-esteem, excessive guilt, self-criticism), self-destructive thoughts, sadness, loss of enjoyment or interest in activities, decreased motivation, apathy, lethargy, irritability, decreased libido, fatigue, and insomnia. The biochemical pathways for depression and energy production are well documented. Without getting too technical, the mood-lifting hormone serotonin is produced in the body by transforming the amino acid tryptophan into serotonin, and vitamin B6 and magnesium are required to do so. Other biochemical deficiencies that are associated with depression are iron deficiency, hypothyroidism, vitamin B12 deficiency, folic acid deficiency, and more.

People with many other conditions may also be suffering from depression. Other conditions with depression as a major component include arthritis, seizure disorder, irritable bowel syndrome (IBS), Lyme disease, migraine headaches, and multiple sclerosis.Many cases of depression have been evaluated and effectively improved with this nutritional biochemical approach. Dr. Neustadt has charted more than 95 percent success rate with depression in his clinic.

Case: Depression / Insomnia / Migraine Headaches

A fifty-two-year-old woman presented to Dr. Neustadt's clinic with a lifelong history of depression. She had had suicidal thoughts as young as five years old, and she attempted suicide once in the past. She also experienced insomnia and occasional migraine headaches.

Her biochemical testing revealed functional deficiencies in nutrients required to generate energy and lift mood. She also complained of difficulty losing weight.

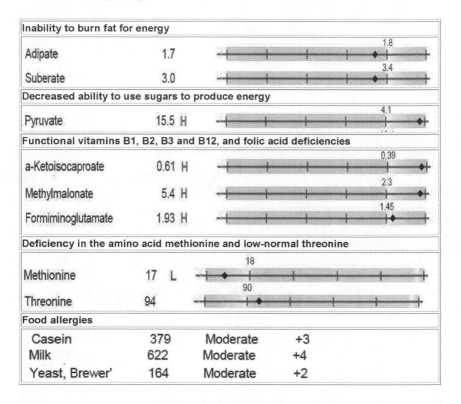

Inability to burn fat for energy			
Adipate	1.7		1.8
Suberate	3.0		3.4
Decreased ability to use sugars to produce energy			
Pyruvate	15.5 H		4.1
Functional vitamins B1, B2, B3 and B12, and folic acid deficiencies			
a-Ketoisocaproate	0.61 H		0.39
Methylmalonate	5.4 H		2.3
Formiminoglutamate	1.93 H		1.45
Deficiency in the amino acid methionine and low-normal threonine			
Methionine	17 L		18
Threonine	94		90
Food allergies			
Casein	379	Moderate	+3
Milk	622	Moderate	+4
Yeast, Brewer'	164	Moderate	+2

She was instructed to avoid the foods she was allergic to, and she was provided with specific dietary recommendations and dietary supplements to give her body the nutrients it was lacking. Two weeks later, at her first follow-up appointment, she reported that she was following the treatment plan diligently, that her mood was "shockingly stable," and that she was not experiencing much depression or anxiety at all. After six weeks on the program, she reported continued improvement in her depression, and that her pants fit looser on her. After three months, she reported complete resolution of her depression for the first time in her life.

Case: Depression / Fatigue / Postnasal Drip / Migraine Headaches / Gas and Bloating / Brain Fog / Postural Hypotension / Weight Gain

A twenty-six-year-old woman presented with a three-year history of depression and fatigue. She also complained that colds would linger longer for her than in others, and that she had postnasal drip almost all the time, premenstrual migraine headaches for the past eight years, abdominal gas/bloating, brain fog, postural hypotension (getting lightheaded when she stood up) "all the time," and an increase in ten pounds of weight in the past couple of years, which she could not lose despite how much she exercised. She rated her energy at three out of ten, with ten being best.

Her MetaCT 400 test results revealed (1) deficiencies in all ten essential amino acids; (2) iron deficiency (low ferritin); (3) multiple mineral deficiencies; (4) elevated free radial damage to cell membranes (elevated lipid peroxides); (5) low vitamin D (risk factor for breast cancer); (6) low omega-6 series fatty acids; (7) functional vitamin deficiencies for energy production; (8) impaired liver detoxification pathways; (9) intestinal bacterial and fungal overgrowth; (10) and severe food intolerances to milk, casein (a protein in milk), and eggs (white and yolk), as well as moderate intolerance to ginger.

Food allergies to dairy, eggs and ginger			
Casein	> 2000	Severe	+5
Egg, White	> 2000	Severe	+5
Egg, Yolk	337	Mod	+3
Milk	> 2000	Severe	+5
Ginger	178	Mod	+3

Amino acid deficiencies

Arginine	49 L	50 - 160	50 — 160
Histidine	68 L	70 - 140	70 — 140
Isoleucine	45 L	50 - 160	50 — 160
Leucine	82 L	90 - 200	90 — 200
Lysine	145 L	150 - 300	150 — 300
Methionine	23 L	25 - 50	25 — 50
Phenylalanine	52	45 - 140	45 — 140
Threonine	93 L	100 - 250	100 — 250
Tryptophan	32 L	35 - 65	35 — 65
Valine	159 L	170 - 420	170 — 420
Tyrosine	43 L	50 - 120	50 — 120

Low minerals		
Chromium	0.28	
Copper	0.59	
Magnesium	43	
Manganese	0.28	
Potassium	1,637	
Selenium	0.16	
Vanadium	0.09 L	
Zinc	6.2	

Low serotonin production (low 5-Hydroxyindoleacetate), associated with depression. Serotonin production requires tryptophan, vitamin B6 and magnesium.

		1.5	5.6
5-Hydroxyindoleacetate	1.8		

Low Coenzyme Q10, a vitamin required for energy production, and an antioxidant

		0.50	1.50
Coenzyme Q10	0.46 L		

Elevated free radical damage to cell membranes

		1.5
Lipid Peroxides	1.8 H	

Vitamin D insufficiency

		16	32
25-hydroxyvitamin D	32		

Low omega-6 series, polyunsaturated fatty acids

		1,303	2,534
Linoleic (18:2n6)	1,144 L		
		4.8	26.1
Gamma Linolenic (18:3n6)	4.2 L		
		6.3	18.8
Eicosadienoic (20:2n6)	5.3 L		
		47	161
Dihomogamma Linolenic (20:3n6)	31 L		

This woman was placed on a comprehensive nutritional medicine program consisting of a combination of diet and nutraceuticals, and it was recommended that she receive counseling. After two weeks on the program, she reported that her energy had already increased, and that she no longer experienced postnasal drip. After six weeks on the program, she reported that her energy had increased to nine out of ten, with ten being best. She had no postnasal drip, no migraine headaches, no abdominal bloating, and she no longer got lightheaded when she stood up (postural hypotension). Her depression had also completely resolved.

Obesity and Diabetes

Obesity is a dangerous metabolic condition that results in increased risk of diabetes, heart disease, cancer, degenerative joint disease, and premature death. Obesity in the United States has increased at an epidemic rate over the last twenty years. The percentage of U.S. adults classified as overweight increased from 56 percent in 1994 to 65 percent in 2002, and obesity increased from 23 percent to 30 percent during this same period. Approximately 16 percent of children and adolescents six to nineteen years old were overweight in 2002.

Obesity is frequently accompanied by diabetes. Diabetes Mellitus (diabetes) is a chronic condition that affects over 19 million Americans. Type 2 diabetes is the most prevalent form, affecting approximately 17 million individuals. The incidence of type 2 diabetes is growing, with a 49 percent increase in diagnoses between 1990 and 2000. Type 2 diabetes used to be called adult-onset diabetes and noninsulin-dependent diabetes mellitus. New evidence has made these terms obsolete, as they are no longer adequately descriptive. This is because with incidence of type 2 diabetes in children skyrocketing, the disease is no longer primarily limited to adults. Additionally, if the condition is not controlled, insulin administration is required in the later stages of disease management. Type 2 diabetes is thought to be preceded by a condition known as insulin resistance syndrome, or metabolic syndrome. This prediabetic state may involve a decrease in the ability of cells to respond to insulin (insulin resistance), a decrease in HDL cholesterol, and an increase in LDL cholesterol, obesity, and high blood pressure.

Case: Obesity / Prediabetes / Fatigue

This is the case of a fifty-five-year-old man who had been struggling for years, spending tens of thousands of dollars on personal trainers and medical testing to improve his health. However, his health continued to deteriorate. He rated his energy at one out of ten (ten being best) and complained of being extremely tired all the time. He wanted to improve his health, but he was too fatigued to exercise. His MetaCT 400 biochemical test panel revealed extremely elevated insulin and fasting blood sugar, inability to produce energy due to deficiencies in nutrients required to burn fats and sugars for energy, a raging intestinal fungal infection (candidiasis), and allergies to eighteen different common foods, such as garlic, eggs, dairy, and almonds. Eating foods one is allergic to causes a chronic inflammation in the gut, which can decrease the ability to digest and absorb nutrients, predispose someone to intestinal infections, cause malnutrition, and set someone up for long-term degenerative diseases such as diabetes and obesity.

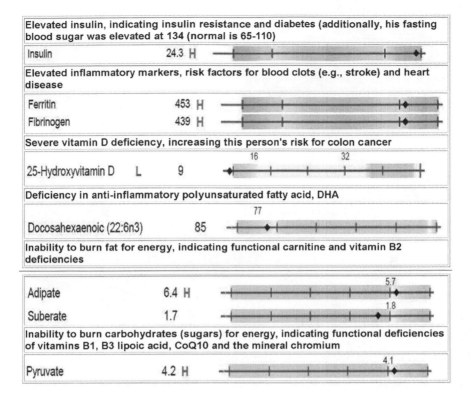

Elevated insulin, indicating insulin resistance and diabetes (additionally, his fasting blood sugar was elevated at 134 (normal is 65-110)

Insulin   24.3 H

Elevated inflammatory markers, risk factors for blood clots (e.g., stroke) and heart disease

Ferritin   453 H

Fibrinogen   439 H

Severe vitamin D deficiency, increasing this person's risk for colon cancer

25-Hydroxyvitamin D   L   9

Deficiency in anti-inflammatory polyunsaturated fatty acid, DHA

Docosahexaenoic (22:6n3)   85

Inability to burn fat for energy, indicating functional carnitine and vitamin B2 deficiencies

Adipate   6.4 H

Suberate   1.7

Inability to burn carbohydrates (sugars) for energy, indicating functional deficiencies of vitamins B1, B3 lipoic acid, CoQ10 and the mineral chromium

Pyruvate   4.2 H

Inability to utilize branched chain amino acids--functional vitamins B1, B2 and B3 deficiency		
a-Ketoisocaproate	0.42 H	0.39 ├────────────┤
Intestinal Fungal Dysbiosis (Candidiasis)		
D-Arabinitol	72 H	32 ├────────────┤

Food Allergies (IgG 90-Antigen Test)			
Casein	> 2000	Severe	+5
Egg, White	> 2000	Severe	+5
Egg, Yolk	147	Mild	+2
Milk	> 2000	Severe	+5
Barley	1,683	Severe	+5
Rye	> 2000	Severe	+5
Wheat	1,882	Severe	+5
Navy Bean	376	Mod	+3
Peanut	> 2000	Severe	+5
Malt	> 2000	Severe	+5
Almond	1,712	Severe	+5
Cashew	> 2000	Severe	+5
Pistachio	> 2000	Severe	+5
Sesame	85	Mild	+2
Sunflower	158	Mod	+3
Garlic	153	Mod	+3
Mustard Greens	1,208	Severe	+5

This gentleman was placed on an aggressive plan of dietary modification, exercise, and dietary supplements to help correct his biochemical abnormalities, decrease his weight, and restore his health. He worked with a nutritionist and exercised regularly. After three months, a retest of his fasting insulin showed that it had decreased by 50 percent (see below), and he had also decreased his waistline by two pant sizes.

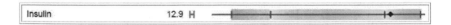

Over time, this person will likely be able to reintroduce some of the foods to which he was allergic, but only after following a gut restoration program intended to rid the intestines of the fungal overgrowth, decrease the inflammation, and heal the cells lining the intestinal tract. However, the message here is that through a simple, customized approach to health care, based on testing the underlying biochemical abnormalities creating the disease, it's quite easy to improve one's health. What people need first, however, are the data to create the plan, which are provided through testing.

Fatigue

Fatigue is a common complaint that has many causes. The underlying biochemistry is that the body is unable to create enough cellular energy, called adenosine triphosphate (ATP), to keep up with the demands. Nutritional deficiencies, infections, cancer, and food allergies can all cause fatigue and other symptoms. People usually do not suffer just from fatigue, but rather fatigue accompanied by depression, muscle aches, joint aches, weight loss or weight gain, abdominal gas and bloating, recurrent upper respiratory or urinary tract infections, and food allergies.

Refer to the following cases in this book where fatigue was one of the major complaints: arthritis, cancer, depression, Lyme disease, overweight/obesity.

Irritable Bowel Syndrome

Irritable Bowel Syndrome (IBS), as the name implies, is a grouping of symptoms that include gas and bloating, abdominal discomfort and constipation or diarrhea. IBS is a diagnosis of exclusion, meaning it is diagnosed after other conditions, such as irritable bowel disease (IBD) has been ruled out. Many natural treatments can help IBS. In one study, meditating fifteen minutes twice daily significantly decreased diarrhea, bloating, flatulence, and belching.[73, 74] Not surprisingly, the study reported no side effects.

Dietary allergies can contribute to IBS symptoms. Eliminating them can lead to dramatic improvement as well. A recent review of dietary allergies in IBS published in *Neurogastroenterology & Motility* concluded that excluding dietary allergens can lead to an improvement in up to 71 percent of IBS sufferers. Blood tests for IgG4 antibodies and the allergy elimination-challenge tests are the most sensitive. In an elimination-challenge test, patients follow a hypoallergenic diet for a prescribed period, while tracking their symptoms in a journal. Then they methodically, and with guidance from a clinician, reintroduce foods one at a time. If symptoms return with specific foods, the patient eliminates them from her diet altogether—perhaps not forever, but for a while.

Case: Irritable Bowel Syndrome / Depression

A forty-nine-year-old woman complained of diarrhea multiple times a week, with a past diagnosis of diarrhea-predominant IBS. She would experience bouts of urgency several times a day, during which she would be forced to stop anything she was doing to rush to the bathroom. She also was experiencing depression for which she was taking 40 mg of Prozac for the depression. Her health goal was to test for the possible underlying causes of her IBS so that she could get rid of it once and for all.

Her MetaCT 400 test results revealed severe allergies to dairy; functional hypothyroidism (low T3); deficiency in all ten essential amino acids and some nonessential amino acids; multiple essential mineral deficiencies (magnesium, zinc, and manganese); elevated free radical damage to lipids and DNA, which are risk factors for heart disease and cancer; mercury toxicity, a risk factor for depression and irritability; vitamin D insufficiency, a risk factor for colorectal cancer, osteoporosis, and cervical cancer; decreased ability to burn fats and carbohydrates for energy production; borderline vitamin B12 deficiency, a risk factor for dementia; intestinal bacterial dysbiosis, a risk factor for malabsorption and nutritional deficiencies; and iron deficiency (low ferritin). These test results explained her IBS and depression (below).

Food allergies, explaining her IBS symptoms			
Casein	1,565	Severe	+5
Milk	1,246	Severe	+5

Note: Casein is a protein found in high concentrations in dairy and dairy products

Intestinal bacterial infection, explaining her IBS symptoms

Indican	116 H	80

Amino acid deficiencies, explaining fatigue, depression, exercise intolerance			
1 Arginine	55	50 - 160	50 — 160
2 Histidine	66 L	70 - 140	70 — 140
3 Isoleucine	33 L	50 - 160	50 — 160
4 Leucine	64 L	90 - 200	90 — 200
5 Lysine	139 L	150 - 300	150 — 300
6 Methionine	20 L	25 - 50	25 — 50
7 Phenylalanine	37 L	45 - 140	45 — 140
8 Threonine	109	100 - 250	100 — 250
9 Tryptophan	28 L	35 - 65	35 — 65
10 Valine	153 L	170 - 420	170 — 420

Low minerals, explaining fatigue, increased free radical damage to DNA		
Magnesium*	19 L	23
Zinc	4.6 L	4.7
Copper	325	311
Manganese	29 L	32

Mercury toxicity		
Mercury	11	4

Elevated free radical damage to cell membranes (lipid peroxides) and to DNA (8-Hydroxy-2-deoxyguanosine)		
Lipid Peroxides	1.9 H	1.5
8-Hydroxy-2-deoxyguanosine	6.7 H	5.3

This woman was placed on a therapeutic elimination diet, her bacterial infection was treated, and her nutritional deficiencies were addressed with dietary supplements and dietary modification. After six weeks of being on the program, her diarrhea had decreased by 80 percent, and she no longer had any urgency. After twelve weeks, her IBS had decreased by 90 percent. She no longer experienced gas/bloating or diarrhea, except when she ate dairy. Her mood had also improved during this period. She reported feeling calmer, and she spoke with her physician about coming going off her antidepressant medication.

Lyme Disease

Lyme disease is an infectious disease caused by spirochete bacteria from the genus *Borrelia*. People can become infected from a deer tick bite and other ticks that carry the disease. Lyme disease can affect all body systems. Symptoms include a rash, flu-like symptoms, muscle pain, joint pain, neurologic symptoms, psychiatric symptoms, and cardiac symptoms.

Case: Lyme Disease / Severe Whole-Body Pain / Muscle Spasms / Depression / Anxiety / Severe Fatigue / Brain Fog

The desperate parents of a twenty-year-old female contacted the clinic to order a comprehensive nutritional biochemistry evaluation for their daughter. She had been suffering for more than eight years with progressively worse and debilitating symptoms. She had severe muscle weakness and spasms to the extent that she would be unable to walk for days. She was in chronic, severe pain all over her body, and she suffered from depression and anxiety. This young woman also experienced severe fatigue and brain fog.

Every organ system was dysfunctional. Although her symptoms predated the diagnosis, she was diagnosed with Lyme disease and was on repeated rounds of oral and intravenous antibiotics for years. She was prescribed multiple antidepressant medications and narcotics, including ever-increasing doses of methadone. All these medical measures were merely symptomatic treatments, and she continued to deteriorate.

Her lab tests revealed deficiencies in almost every category of nutrients (amino acids, vitamins, and minerals) and biochemical pathways. In short, her entire biochemistry was not working properly. This extreme and rare situation is what the authors of this book have called *total body breakdown*, which they suspect underlies the following medical

131

diagnoses—Lyme disease, chronic fatigue syndrome, hypopituitaryism, and mitochondrial disease.

Amino acid deficiencies			
Arginine	46 L	50 - 160	
Histidine	72	70 - 140	
Isoleucine	57	50 - 160	
Leucine	82 L	90 - 200	
Lysine	135 L	150 - 300	
Methionine	26	25 - 50	
Phenylalanine	46	45 - 140	
Tryptophan	34 L	35 - 65	
Valine	173	170 - 420	
Glycine	138 L	225 - 450	
Serine	94	90 - 210	
Taurine	68	50 - 250	
Tyrosine	43 L	50 - 120	
Glutamine	537 L	600 - 1,050	
Iron-deficiency anemia			
Ferritin	4 L		

Inflammation		
c-Reactive Protein (HS)	3.7 H	
Insulin resistance		

Insulin	11.6	
Deficient essential minerals		
Chromium	0.24 L	
Copper	0.52	
Magnesium	31 L	
Manganese	0.31	
Selenium	0.13	
Vanadium	0.10	
Zinc	6.5	
Elevated toxic metal		
Arsenic	0.018	
Low antioxidants		
Coenzyme Q10	0.52	0.50 — 1.50
Vitamin E	9.1	8.6 — 24.6
Decreased ability to burn fats for energy		
Adipate	1.8	1.8
Suberate	9.1 H	3.4
Decreased ability to burn carbohydrates for energy		
Lactate	16.9	19.4
Low B-complex vitamins and biotin		
a-Keto-ß-Methylvalerate	1.9 H	1.6
Xanthurenate	0.85 H	0.70
ß-Hydroxyisovalerate	12.9 H	9.0

Neurotransmitter imbalances (low epinephrine, elevated dopamine)		
Vanilmandelate	1.7 L	1.9 — 4.8
Homovanillate	8.4 H	2.2 — 8.3
Intestinal bacterial overgrowth		
Phenylpropionate	3.3 H	2.1
p-Hydroxybenzoate	1.3 H	1.0
p-Hydroxyphenylacetate	18 H	15
Tricarballylate	1.7 H	1.6

This complicated case required close management and a complex plan. Follow-up telephone consultations occurred weekly, and modifications to the plan were made as appropriate and necessary. She was placed on a comprehensive antibacterial, antifungal, and gut-rebuilding protocol for intestinal health. She began taking appropriate amino acids, vitamins, minerals, and antioxidants. This woman was also counseled on not pushing herself too hard, so that as she began to feel better, she would allow her body to heal without putting additional stress on her body systems.

She progressively began to improve, and after two weeks, her mother reported that at times she had her daughter back. As the weeks went on, the young woman continued to improve. She reported increased energy, improved mental acuity, decreased pain, a lifting of her depression, and a cessation of headaches. Her mother reported that it became easier to wake her daughter in the morning and after she took a nap, and that her daughter began getting herself out of bed in the morning and off to school without the need for assistance. She was able to resume some normal activities, even ice-skating, as well as attend college.

Migraine Headaches

Migraine headaches can cause debilitating pain so severe that relief is only obtained by lying down in a dark, quiet place. Migraine afflicts 28 million Americans, with females suffering more frequently (17 percent) than males (6 percent). The pain usually is on one side of the head, although about a third of the time the pain is on both sides. People suffering from migraines may also experience nausea, vomiting, diarrhea, cold hands, cold feet, and sensitivity to both light and sound. Typically, attacks can last from four to seventy-two hours.

Case: Migraine Headache / Depression / Premenstrual Syndrome

A twenty-three-year-old woman had been suffering for seven years with migraine headaches. Up until one year ago she had been getting migraine headaches three times each year; however, the frequency had increased and she suffered migraine headaches daily now. Her migraines were accompanies by visual disturbances that manifested as pain and seeing "little stars all over." A careful medical history revealed that her migraine headaches began when she was in high school and suffering from anorexia nervosa and intense periods of exercise. She had also been experiencing depression and fatigue. Given her medical history and chief complaint of migraine headaches, she was at high risk for underlying nutritional deficiencies.

When she was evaluated, she was taking three different medications for migraine headaches—Relpax, Zanaflex, and Ultracet—and Fuoxetine (Prozac), an antidepressant medication. This woman also suffered from painful periods (dysmenorrhea) for which she had to take Tylenol. One day prior to each period, she would become so emotional that she would break down in tears, and she stated that her mood was quite erratic.

Her biochemical testing revealed the underlying causes for her symptoms. She had severe amino acid deficiencies; food allergies; functional deficiencies in B-complex vitamins, of which the most severe was vitamin B6; functional deficiency in carnitine (elevated adipate), meaning that she was having difficulty burning her fats for cellular energy; liver detoxification pathway impairment (elevated orotate); and food allergies for dairy and eggs.

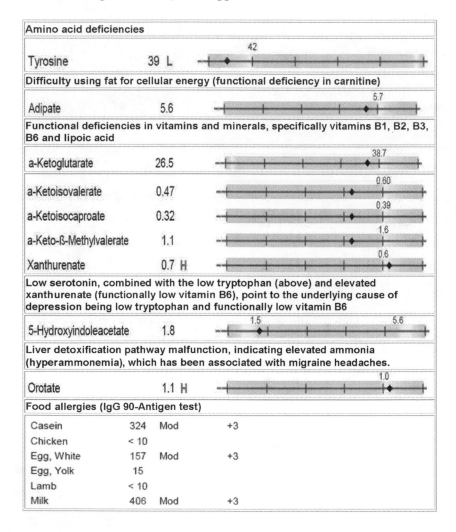

She was placed on a therapeutic diet with specific nutrients to replete her deficiencies. After two weeks on her therapeutic diet and nutraceuticals, she reported a 60 percent improvement in the intensity of her migraine headaches. Additionally, whereas she was experiencing migraines daily before, she had only experienced one migraine in the past two weeks. She could resume her daily activities without any interference from the migraines, and the flashes of light had also improved. With respect to her mood, she stated that her mood was "a lot better; more stable," and her premenstrual syndrome had completely resolved.

After being on the program for six weeks, she continued to experience improvements in her symptoms. She had only experienced one migraine in the previous month since her last appointment, and that was after traveling and eating foods to which she was allergic. She also stated that her depression had completely resolved, and she requested that Dr. Neustadt begin weaning her off her antidepressant medications. After twelve weeks, she reported no migraine headaches, no PMS, and said that her mood was "excellent."

Multiple Sclerosis

Multiple sclerosis (MS) is a neurodegenerative disorder in which the myelin sheath (the layer of fat insulating nerves) in the central nervous system breaks down. Multiple sclerosis is considered an "idiopathic" disease in medicine, meaning that researchers still do not know what causes it. However, much research has been done on the underlying biochemical abnormalities in multiple sclerosis, and advanced testing and a nutritional biochemical approach to treating them have helped people return to good health. Studies have shown a connection between low vitamin D status and MS, low essential fatty acids and MS, and inflammation.

Case: Multiple Sclerosis / Depression

A twenty-five-year-old male presented with MS and a ten-year history of depression. He had been diagnosed with MS two months prior, and he was just completing a round of corticosteroid therapy for the MS symptoms, which included unilateral (one-sided) temporary blindness and incoordination in both legs.

Analyte	Value		Range
Arginine	71		50 - 160
Histidine	54	L	70 - 140
Isoleucine	58		50 - 160
Leucine	101		90 - 200
Lysine	164		150 - 300
Methionine	20	L	25 - 50
Phenylalanine	41	L	45 - 140
Threonine	125		100 - 250
Tryptophan	30	L	35 - 65
Valine	182		170 - 420
Phosphoethanolamine	71	H	<= 30
Fibrinogen	401	H	
Chromium	0.31		
Vanadium	0.11		
Zinc	5.8	L	
Vitamin E	9.8		
Vitamin A	0.56		
25-hydroxyvitamin D	L	15	
Alpha Linolenic (18:3n3)	3.3		
Eicosapentaenoic (20:5n3)	15		
Docosapentaenoic (22:5n3)	64		
Docosahexaenoic (22:6n3)	125		

139

Seizure Disorder / Depression

Case: Seizures / Depression / Fatigue

A thirty-seven-year-old male presented with seizures, lifelong depression, suicidal tendencies, and extreme fatigue. This man was literally at death's doorstep—he was exhausted, unable to care for himself, and without hope. His seizures began four months earlier while on a pleasure trip to Las Vegas. He had no history of head trauma or previous seizure activity. A neurologist evaluated him, ordering a computer tomography (CT) scan, a magnetic resonance imaging (MRI) study, and an electroencephalogram (EEG). All these studies were appropriate for the medical model, and Dr. Neustadt would have ordered them all as well; however, the crucial difference between the nutritional biochemistry approach and that of a well-educated conventional neurologist is that Dr. Neustadt also ordered a comprehensive nutritional biochemistry evaluation.

None of the conventional imaging ordered by the neurologist revealed any abnormalities. The patient was diagnosed as having "pseudoseizures" (literally, "false seizures"), yet there was nothing false about them. The patient was prescribed different antiseizure medications, but none reduced his seizure symptoms at all. Instead, he developed increasing depression because he felt more and more helpless and hopeless because none of his symptoms were relieved after seeing these medical experts.

When he finally arrived at Montana Integrative Medicine and took the comprehensive nutritional biochemistry test, his results explained the underlying causes of all his symptoms. His depression was a result of low epinephrine, low serotonin, low omega-3 fatty acids, and a functional vitamin B6 deficiency. His seizures were due to low phenylalanine, low tyrosine, low dopamine, and functionally low vitamin B6, which is required for dopamine formation. Low dopamine causes seizures and is an underlying cause of Parkinson's disease. Additionally, his medical evaluation, which included a diet recall, made it apparent that the timing of his seizures appeared to coincide with possible low blood sugar, which is documented to cause seizures.

Low essential fatty acids of the omega-3 series		
Alpha Linolenic (18:3n3)	12 L	14
Eicosapentaenoic (20:5n3)	7 L	15
Docosapentaenoic (22:5n3)	21	19
Docosahexaenoic (22:6n3)	51 L	77
Functional vitamin B6 deficiency		
Xanthurenate	0.70	0.70
Neurotransmitter imbalances, with low dopamine (homovanillate)		
Vanilmandelate	1.6 L	1.9 ... 4.8
Homovanillate	1.1 L	2.2 ... 8.3
5-Hydroxyindoleacetate	2.0	1.5 ... 5.6

He was placed on a comprehensive treatment plan that included nutritional cofactors to correct his underlying biochemical dysfunction, as well as a medically directed diet to better control his blood sugar. He was prescribed amino acids, high-dose B vitamins, essential fatty acids, a high-quality multivitamin and mineral supplement, and a high-fiber diet. The patient's seizures stopped after being on the program for four days, and he continued to be seizure free at the three-month follow-up appointment. He also reported no more depression, increased energy, no suicidal thoughts, and feeling better than he could ever remember feeling.

How to Contact Us and Order Tests

Testing kits are shipped all over the world. Here's how it works. When someone is interested in ordering a test, they first complete a Consent for Coaching form, e-mailed, faxed, or mailed to him or her by Dr. Neustadt's staff at Montana Integrative Medicine. When that form is returned to the clinic, the testing kit is shipped to the client. If the test ordered only requires a finger prick blood sample, urine sample, or stool sample, the client collects the specimen and ships it to the lab using a prepaid FedEx envelope. If a blood draw is required, Dr. Neustadt or his staff will find a facility near you to collect the blood, process it, and ship it to the lab. Dr. Neustadt has already established a network of facilities in the United States, so it's likely that there is a convenient blood draw facility near you.

All tests can be ordered through the authors' testing and consulting company:

NBI Testing and Consulting Corporation
1087 Stoneridge Drive, Suite 1
Bozeman, MT 59718
Tel: 800-624-1416
www.nbitesting.com.

To learn more about Dr. John Neustadt's clinical work, go to his website: **www.montanaim.com**.

About the Authors

John Neustadt, ND, received his naturopathic medical degree from Bastyr University. Dr. Neustadt also earned degrees in literature (cum laude) from the University of California, San Diego, and botany (departmental honors) from the University of Washington. He worked as a journalist in Chile and San Francisco before returning to naturopathic medical school. He is medical director of Montana Integrative Medicine and president and CEO of Nutritional Biochemistry, Incorporated (NBI) and NBI Testing and Consulting Corporation in Bozeman, Montana. *Dr. Neustadt is an* editor of the textbook *Laboratory Evaluations for Integrative and Functional Medicine*, is a Contributing Editor to the *Journal of Prolotherapy* and on the editorial advisory board for *Remedies Magazine*. He has published more than one hundred research reviews, is coauthor with Jonathan Wright, MD, of the book *Thriving through Dialysis,* and with Steve Pieczenik, MD, PhD of the book, *A Revolution in Health through Nutritional Biochemistry.*

Steve Pieczenik, MD, PhD, trained in Psychiatry at Harvard and has both an MD from Cornell University Medical College and a PhD in international relations from MIT. He is a board-certified Psychiatrist and was a board examiner in Psychiatry and Neurology. He is chairman of the boards of NBI and NBI Testing and Consulting Corporation, as well as an angel investor who has started more than thirty successful companies.

References

1. Glade MJ. Food, nutrition, and the prevention of cancer: a global perspective. American Institute for Cancer Research/World Cancer Research Fund, American Institute for Cancer Research, 1997. *Nutrition.* Jun 1999;15(6):523-526.

2. *U.S. Department of Health and Human Services. Healthy People 2010: Understanding and Improving Health.* 2d ed. Washington, D.C.: U.S. Government Printing Office; 2000.

3. Jansson ET. Aluminum exposure and Alzheimer's disease. *J Alzheimers Dis.* Dec 2001;3(6):541-549.

4. *Children in the New Millenium. Environmental Impact on Health*: United Nations Environmental Program, United Nations Children's Fund, and World Health Organization; 2002.

5. Mohseni S. Hypoglycemic neuropathy. *Acta Neuropathol (Berl).* Nov 2001;102(5):413-421.

6. Initial sequencing and analysis of the human genome. 2001/02/15/print 2001;409(6822):860-921.

7. Wiemann S, Weil B, Wellenreuther R, et al. Toward a Catalog of Human Genes and Proteins: Sequencing and Analysis of 500 Novel Complete Protein Coding Human cDNAs. *Genome Res.* 2001;11(3):422-435.

8. Rock CL, Lampe JW, Patterson RE. Nutrition, Genetics, and Risks of Cancer. *Annual Review of Public Health.* 2000;21(1):47-64.

9. Muti P, Bradlow HL, Micheli A, et al. Estrogen metabolism and risk of breast cancer: a prospective study of the 2:16alpha-hydroxyestrone ratio in premenopausal and postmenopausal women. *Epidemiology.* Nov 2000;11(6):635-640.

10. Dalessandri KM, Firestone GL, Fitch MD, Bradlow HL, Bjeldanes LF. Pilot Study: Effect of 3,3'-Diindolylmethane Supplements on Urinary Hormone Metabolites in Postmenopausal Women With a History of Early-Stage Breast Cancer. *Nutrition and Cancer.* 2004;50(2):161-167.

11. Gershon M. *The Second Brain: A Groundbreaking New Understanding of Nervous Disorders of the Stomach and Intestine.* New York: Harper Paperbacks; 1999.

12. Saavedra JM, Tschernia A. Human studies with probiotics and prebiotics: clinical implications. *Br J Nutr.* May 2002;87 Suppl 2:S241-246.

13. Bengmark S. Immunonutrition: role of biosurfactants, fiber, and probiotic bacteria. *Nutrition.* Jul-Aug 1998;14(7-8):585-594.

14. Kirjavainen PV, Gibson GR. Healthy gut microflora and allergy: factors influencing development of the microbiota. *Ann Med.* Aug 1999;31(4):288-292.

15. Barbeau WE. Interactions between dietary proteins and the human system: implications for oral tolerance and food-related diseases. *Adv Exp Med Biol.* 1997;415:183-193.

16. Stanley S. Oral tolerance of food. *Curr Allergy Asthma Rep.* Jan 2002;2(1):73-77.

17. Schneeman BO. Gastrointestinal physiology and functions. *Br J Nutr.* Nov 2002;88 Suppl 2:S159-163.

18. Hurwitz A, Brady DA, Schaal SE, Samloff IM, Dedon J, Ruhl CE. Gastric acidity in older adults. *Jama.* Aug 27 1997;278(8):659-662.

19. Kassarjian Z, Russell RM. Hypochlorhydria: A Factor in Nutrition. *Annual Review of Nutrition.* 1989;9(1):271-285.

20. Wood RJ, Suter PM, Russell RM. Mineral requirements of elderly people. *Am J Clin Nutr.* 1995;62(3):493-505.

21. Baik HW, Russell RM. Vitamin B12 deficiency in the elderly. *Annu Rev Nutr.* 1999;19:357-377.

22. Prousky JE. Cobalamin deficiency in elderly patients. *CMAJ.* 2005;172(4):450-a-451.

23. Sturniolo GC, Montino MC, Rossetto L, et al. Inhibition of gastric acid secretion reduces zinc absorption in man. *J Am Coll Nutr.* Aug 1991;10(4):372-375.

24. Kelly GS. Hydrochloric Acid: Physiological Functions and Clinical Implications. *Alt Med Rev.* 1997;2(2):116-127.

25. Sharp GS. The diagnosis and treatment of achlorhydria; preliminary report of new simplified methods. *West J Surg Obstet Gynecol.* Jul 1953;61(7):353-360.

26. Yang YX, Lewis JD, Epstein S, Metz DC. Long-term proton pump inhibitor therapy and risk of hip fracture. *JAMA.* 2006;296(24):2947-2953.

27. Martinsen TC, Bergh K, Waldum HL. Gastric juice: a barrier against infectious diseases. *Basic Clin Pharmacol Toxicol.* Feb 2005;96(2):94-102.

28. Hongo M, Ishimori A, Nagasaki A, Sato T. Effect of duodenal acidification on the lower esophageal sphincter pressure in the dog with special reference to related gastrointestinal hormones. *Tohoku J Exp Med.* Jul 1980;131(3):215-219.

29. Wright JV. *Dr. Wright's Guide to Healing with Nutrition.* New Canaan, CT: Keats Publishing; 1990.

30. Simon GL, Gorbach SL. Intestinal flora in health and disease. *Gastroenterology.* Jan 1984;86(1):174-193.

31. Guarner F, Malagelada J-R. Gut flora in health and disease. *The Lancet.* 2003;361(9356):512-519.

32. Bengmark S. Ecological control of the gastrointestinal tract. The role of probiotic flora. *Gut.* Jan 1998;42(1):2-7.

33. Bralley J, Lord R. *Laboratory Evaluations in Molecular Medicine: Nutrients, Toxicants, and Cell Regulators.* Norcross, GA: The Institute for Advances in Molecular Medicine; 2001.

34. Urita Y, Sugimoto M, Hike K, et al. High incidence of fermentation in the digestive tract in patients with reflux oesophagitis. *Eur J Gastroenterol Hepatol.* May 2006;18(5):531-535.

35. Tomohiko S, Masaki I, Nobue H, Yoko H, Masuo N, Susumu T. Gastric Acid Normosecretion Is Not Essential in the Pathogenesis of Mild Erosive Gastroesophageal Reflux Disease

in Relation to Helicobacter pylori Status. *Digestive Diseases and Sciences.* 2004;V49(5):787-794.

36. Bralley J, Lord R. Chapter 4: Amino Acids. *Laboratory Evaluations in Molecular Medicine: Nutrients, Toxicants, and Cell Regulators.* Norcross, GA: The Institute for Advances in Molecular Medicine; 2001:75-131.

37. Santos J, Bayarri C, Saperas E, et al. Characterisation of immune mediator release during the immediate response to segmental mucosal challenge in the jejunum of patients with food allergy. *Gut.* 1999;45(4):553-558.

38. Rodrigo L. Celiac disease. *World J Gastroenterol.* Nov 7 2006;12(41):6585-6593.

39. Hernandez L, Green PH. Extraintestinal manifestations of celiac disease. *Curr Gastroenterol Rep.* Oct 2006;8(5):383-389.

40. Hvatum M, Kanerud L, Hallgren R, Brandtzaeg P. The gut-joint axis: cross reactive food antibodies in rheumatoid arthritis. *Gut.* 2006;55(9):1240-1247.

41. Zar S, Kumar D, Benson MJ. Food hypersensitivity and irritable bowel syndrome. *Alimentary Pharmacology & Therapeutics.* 2001;15(4):439-449.

42. Rowntree S, Platts-Mills TA, Cogswell JJ, Mitchell EB. A subclass IgG4-specific antigen-binding radioimmunoassay (RIA): comparison between IgG and IgG4 antibodies to food and inhaled antigens in adult atopic dermatitis after desensitization treatment and during development of antibody responses in children. *J Allergy Clin Immunol.* Oct 1987;80(4):622-630.

43. Calkhoven PG, Aalbers M, Koshte VL, et al. Relationship between IgG1 and IgG4 antibodies to foods and the development of IgE antibodies to inhalant allergens. II. Increased levels of IgG antibodies to foods in children who subsequently develop IgE antibodies to inhalant allergens. *Clin Exp Allergy.* Jan 1991;21(1):99-107.

44. Johnson M, Fischer J. Role of minerals on protecting against free radicals. *Food Tech.* May 1994:112-120.

45. Kitts D. An evaluation of the multiple effects of the antioxidant vitamins. *Trends Food Sci Tech.* 1997;8:198-203.

46. Zamora R, Hidalgo F, Tappel A. Comparative antioxidant effectiveness of dietary b-carotene, Vitamin E, Selenium and Coenzyme Q10 in rat erythrocytes and plasma. *J Nutr.* 1991;121:50-56.

47. Pantuck EJ, Pantuck CB, Garland WA, et al. Stimulatory effect of brussels sprouts and cabbage on human drug metabolism. *Clin Pharmacol Ther.* Jan 1979;25(1):88-95.

48. Ip C, Lisk DJ. Modulation of phase I and phase II xenobiotic-metabolizing enzymes by selenium-enriched garlic in rats. *Nutr Cancer.* 1997;28(2):184-188.

49. Appelt LC, Reicks MM. Soy feeding induces phase II enzymes in rat tissues. *Nutr Cancer.* 1997;28(3):270-275.

50. Barch DH, Rundhaugen LM, Pillay NS. Ellagic acid induces transcription of the rat glutathione S-transferase-Ya gene. *Carcinogenesis.* Mar 1995;16(3):665-668.

51. Li Y, Wang E, Patten CJ, Chen L, Yang CS. Effects of flavonoids on cytochrome P450-dependent acetaminophen metabolism in rats and human liver microsomes. *Drug Metab Dispos.* Jul-Aug 1994;22(4):566-571.

52. Maltzman TH, Christou M, Gould MN, Jefcoate CR. Effects of monoterpenoids on in vivo DMBA-DNA adduct formation and on phase I hepatic metabolizing enzymes. *Carcinogenesis.* Nov 1991;12(11):2081-2087.

53. Miller EC, Miller JA. Searches for ultimate chemical carcinogens and their reactions with cellular macromolecules. *Cancer.* May 15 1981;47(10):2327-2345.

54. Larson EB, Wang L, Bowen JD, et al. Exercise Is Associated with Reduced Risk for Incident Dementia among Persons 65 Years of Age and Older. *Ann Intern Med.* 2006;144(2):73-81.

55. Leitzmann MF, Park Y, Blair A, et al. Physical activity recommendations and decreased risk of mortality. *Arch Intern Med.* Dec 10 2007;167(22):2453-2460.

56. Oberg E. Physical Activity Prescription: Our Best Medicine. *Integr Med.* 2007;6(5):18-22.

57. Wurtman RJ, Wurtman JJ. Brain serotonin, carbohydrate-craving, obesity and depression. *Obes Res.* Nov 1995;3 Suppl 4:477S-480S.

58. Garrod AE. The incidence of alkaptonuria: a study in chemical individuality. *Lancet.* 1902;11:1616-1620.

59. Williams R. *Biochemical Individuality: the basis for the genotrophic concept.* New York: McGraw-Hill; 1998.

60. Ames BN, Elson-Schwab I, Silver EA. High-dose vitamin therapy stimulates variant enzymes with decreased coenzyme binding affinity (increased K(m)): relevance to genetic disease and polymorphisms. *Am J Clin Nutr.* Apr 2002;75(4):616-658.

61. Ames BN. The metabolic tune-up: metabolic harmony and disease prevention. *J Nutr.* May 2003;133(5 Suppl 1):1544S-1548S.

62. Ames BN, Liu J. Delaying the Mitochondrial Decay of Aging with Acetylcarnitine. Vol 1033; 2004:108-116.

63. Ames BN, Shigenaga MK, Hagen TM. Oxidants, antioxidants, and the degenerative diseases of aging. *Proc Natl Acad Sci U S A.* Sep 1 1993;90(17):7915-7922.

64. EC 1.14.16.1. http://www.chem.qmul.ac.uk/iubmb/enzyme/EC1/14/16/1.html. Accessed February 27, 2007.

65. Seashore MR. Tetrahydrobiopterin and Dietary Restriction in Mild Phenylketonuria. *N Engl J Med.* 2002;347(26):2094-2095.

66. Muntau AC, Roschinger W, Habich M, et al. Tetrahydrobiopterin as an Alternative Treatment for Mild Phenylketonuria. *N Engl J Med.* 2002;347(26):2122-2132.

67. Kure S, Hou D-C, Ohura T, et al. Tetrahydrobiopterin-responsive phenylalanine hydroxylase deficiency. *The Journal of Pediatrics.* 1999;135(3):375-378.

68. Rose WC, Haines WJ, Warner DT. The amino acid requirements of man. V. The role of lysine, arginine, and tryptophan. *J Biol Chem.* Jan 1954;206(1):421-430.

69. Rose WC, Warner DT, Haines WJ. The amino acid requirements of man. IV. The role of leucine and phenylalanine. *J Biol Chem.* Dec 1951;193(2):613-620.

70. Rose WC, Haines WJ, Warner DT. The amino acid requirements of man. III. The role of isoleucine; additional evidence concerning histidine. *J Biol Chem.* Dec 1951;193(2):605-612.

71. Rose WC, Haines WJ, Warner DT, Johnson JE. The amino acid requirements of man. II. The role of threonine and histidine. *J Biol Chem.* Jan 1951;188(1):49-58.

72. Saltzman JR, Russell RM. The aging gut. Nutritional issues. *Gastroenterol Clin North Am.* Jun 1998;27(2):309-324.

73. Keefer L, Blanchard EB. The effects of relaxation response meditation on the symptoms of irritable bowel syndrome: results of a controlled treatment study. *Behav Res Ther.* Jul 2001;39(7):801-811.

74. Keefer L, Blanchard EB. A one year follow-up of relaxation response meditation as a treatment for irritable bowel syndrome. *Behav Res Ther.* May 2002;40(5):541-546.

INDEX

The *t* after page numbers indicates text in a table.

A

abdominal gas
  cases about, 85–92, 117–120, 126, 127
  causes of, 33
  and food allergies, 72
  and IgG reactions, 35, 73
  and intestinal candidiasis, 2
  and intestinal dysbiosis, 32
  and parasitic infections, 75, 76*t*
acetaminophen, 54
aches. *See* joint aches and pain; muscles
achlorhydria, 31
acid-blocking medications, 32, 33
Aciphex, 31
acute spasm of the bronchi, 58–59
Adderrall, 102
adenosine triphosphate (ATP), 126
ADHD (Attention Deficit Hyperactivity Disorder), 102–103
adrenal fatigue, 52
adult-onset diabetes. *See* type 2 diabetes
aerobic exercises, 59
African American men, and prostate cancer, 22
age-related degeneration (ARD), 85–92
alcohol, 12, 13, 31
allergies
  bee stings, 35, 73
  food. *See* food allergies

  peanuts, 35, 73
alpha lipoic acid, 10, 40
aluminum, 2
Alzheimer's disease, 2
Ames, Bruce, 69
amino acid powder, customized, 88, 92
amino acid profile
  sample test results, 87*t*, 90*t*, 94*t*, 97*t*, 105*t*, 109*t*, 113*t*, 118*t*, 129*t*, 132*t*, 136*t*, 139*t*
  as variable on MetaCT™ Test, 65*t*
anemia, 40
anorexia nervosa, 135
antibody, 35, 73
antibody-antigen complexes, 35, 73–74
antidepressants, 8, 9–10, 11, 54, 131, 135
antigen, 35, 73
antioxidants, 43, 94*t*, 133*t*
anxiety, 40*t*, 131–134
apples, 81
Archives of Internal Medicine, 57
ARD (age-related degeneration), 85–92
arsenic, 2
arthritis, 13, 93–98
Asian/Pacific Islanders, and prostate cancer, 22
asthma, 13, 99–101. *See also* exertion asthma
ATP (adenosine triphosphate), 126
Attention Deficit Hyperactivity Disorder (ADHD), 102–103
autoimmune diseases, 23*t*
Axid, 31

B

fatty acid profile
  sample test results, 95t, 97t, 105t, 110t, 119t, 141t
  as variable on MetaCT™ Test, 66t
FDA (Food and Drug Administration), 40, 79, 81
Federal Council on Environmental Quality, 47
fight-or-flight response, 36, 37–38
fish, and toxic metals, 39, 79, 80
flame retardants, 45
flatulence. See abdominal gas
flavonoids, 55t
flexible sigmoidoscopy, 17t, 24t, 25t
Focalin, 102
folic acid, 55t, 88t, 98t
food. See also specific food items
  dairy, 22, 80
  and detoxification, 55t
  fats, 80
  fruits, 43–44, 55t, 80–81, 82–83
  organic, 79–83
  protein, 35, 39, 55t, 73, 79, 80
  vegetables, 21, 55t, 81–82, 83
food allergies. See also Celiac disease
  cases about, 85, 102
  elimination-challenge tests, 127
  results of, 31, 34, 35
  sample test results, 88t, 92t, 95t, 110t, 113t, 116t, 118t, 123t, 129t, 136t
  and stress, 36
  symptoms of, 72, 73
Food and Drug Administration (FDA), 40, 79, 81
food intolerances. See food allergies
free radical damage
  cases about, 94t, 113t, 119t, 129t
  and fight-or-flight situation, 38
  markers of inflammation test, 65t
fullness, prolonged sense of, 32
fungi, 32, 33, 43
fungicides, 43, 81
Fuoxetine (Prozac), 135

G

GALT (gut-associated lymph tissue), 30
garlic, 55t
Garrod, Archibald E., 68–69
gas. See abdominal gas
gastric reflux, 33, 34
gastroesophageal reflux disorder (GERD), 33, 34
gastrointerstinal microbial ecology profile, 75–77
gastrointestinal microbiology profile, 65t
gene-nutrient interactions, 70
genes, as protein creators, 18
genetics
  and breast cancer, 20
  vs. lifestyle, 1, 23
  as predisposition to disease, 18
genetrophic approach, 69
GERD (gastroesophageal reflux disorder), 33, 34
glaucoma screening, 17t, 24t, 25t
gluten, 34
grape skin, 55t
grapes, 82–83
green bell peppers, 83
guiac test, 17t, 24t, 33, 75
gut. See also stomach acid production
  health of, 28
  hyperpermeable gut, 36
  restoration of, 92, 95, 123–124
gut-associated lymph tissue (GALT), 30

H

hair loss, 32, 40t
HDL cholesterol, 57, 121
health. See also patients
  defined, 1–3, 27
  managing your own, 9
  and mindset, 27
  program, customized, 11, 79–84
hearing test, 24t
heart disease, 1, 23t, 38
heartburn, 32

Heidelburg pH capsule test, 34
Helicobacter pylori (H. pylori) infection, 34, 77
herbicides, 43
Herceptin, 107
high-risk patients, 18, 23, 24*t*
hip fractures, 32
histidine, 33, 34
holistic treatment, 8
homocysteine test, 24*t*
hormones and neurotransmitter markers, 66*t*
hydrochloric acid capsules, 34
hydroxyestrogen ratio, 20, 21
hyperpermeable gut, 36
hypersensitivity reactions, 35, 73
hypochlorhydria, 31
hypoglycemia, 12, 13
hypopituitaryism, 132

I

IBD (inflammatory bowel disease), 112
IBD (irritable bowel disease), 127
IBS (irritable bowel syndrome), 33, 127–130
IgA, 73
IgE, 35, 73
IgG, 34–35, 67*t*, 73, 99
IgG4 antibody tests, 127
IgM, 73
immediate hypersensitivity reactions, 35, 73
immune system, 27, 30, 36
immunoglobulin, 72–73
indigestion, 32, 108–111
inducible pathway, 21
inflammation, 133*t*
inflammatory bowel disease (IBD), 112
inflammatory markers, 24*t*, 123*t*
insecticides, 43
insomnia
    and age-related degeneration (ARD), 85

cases about, 96–98, 108–111, 112, 115–116
    and hypoglycemia, 12
    as symptom of mercury toxicity, 40*t*
insulin
    defined, 12
    resistance, 60–61, 121, 133*t*
    sample test results, 100*t*, 123*t*
    test, 24*t*, 97*t*
intelligence quotient (IQ), and mercury toxicity, 40*t*
intestinal bacterial overgrowth, 88*t*, 92*t*, 134*t*
intestinal candidiasis, 2
intestinal dysbiosis, 2, 31, 32–33, 85, 113*t*
intestinal fungal dysbiosis, 124*t*
intestinal fungal overgrowth, 88*t*, 92*t*
intestinal infections, 100*t*, 102–103, 110*t*, 129*t*
intestines, 30, 34, 36–37
intracellular magnesium test, 24*t*
iron, 40, 55*t*, 64*t*, 132*t*
irritable bowel disease (IBD), 127
irritable bowel syndrome (IBS), 13, 127–130
ischemia, 59

J

joint aches and pain, 35, 36, 73, 93–95, 96–98

K

kava kava, 104
kohlrabi, 21, 55*t*
Kraepelin, Emil, 104

L

laboratory tests. *See* biochemical tests
Lancer, 68
L-carnitine, 40, 107, 110*t*
LDL cholesterol, 57, 121
lean body mass measurement, 17*t*, 24*t*
Lexapro, 8, 11

minerals
  and detoxification, 55t
  intracellular essential, 64t
mitochondrial disease, 132
moles, 17t, 25t
Montana Integrative Medicine (MIM), 7, 143
MRI (magnetic resonance imaging), 140
multiple sclerosis (MS), 138–139
muscles, 28, 40, 86–89, 93–95, 108–111, 131–134
musculoskeletal system, 28

N

National Academy of Sciences, 48
National Library of Medicine, 29
natural methods, 29
naturopathic medicine, 6
NBI (Nutritional Biochemistry, Inc.), 7, 143
NBI Testing and Consulting Corp. (NBITC), 7, 143
nectarines, 82
nervous system, 37–38
Neurogastroenterology & Motility, 127
neurological system, 27
neuropathy, diabetic peripheral, 40
neurotoxins, 81
neurotransmitter imbalances, 134t, 141t
neurotransmitter markers and hormones, 66t
New England Journal of Medicine, 9
Nexium, 31
noninsulin-dependent diabetes mellitus. *See* type 2 diabetes
non-vitamin nutrients, and detoxification, 55t
norepinephrine, 36, 100
nutraceuticals, 40, 68
nutrients, 10, 11, 55t
nutrition
  and detoxification, 54, 55t
  and severe genetic conditions, 71

nutritional biochemistry, 5, 63, 68, 77. *See also* biochemical tests
Nutritional Biochemistry, Inc. (NBI), 7, 143

O

O&Px3 (ova & parasite) test, 75
obesity, 13, 38, 61, 62, 121–125
organic foods, recommended to buy, 79–83
osteoporosis, 38
overweight, and insulin resistance, 60–61
oxygen, as nutrient, 83

P

PAH (phenylalanine hydroxylase), 70
pain
  joint, 35, 36, 73, 93–95, 96–98
  muscle, 86–89, 93–95
  whole-body, 131–134
The Pants Test, 60
pap smear, 17t, 24t, 25t
parabens exposure, and breast cancer, 3
parasitic infections, symptoms of, 76t–77t
parasympathetic nervous system, 37
patients
  advocacy of self, 8, 21, 25
  and changes, meaningful, 21
  and diagnosis vs. underlying causes, 13
  family history, 18, 79
  high-risk, 18, 23, 24t
  low-risk, 17t
  medical history, 2
  and physician visits, 19, 28
  rationalizations by, 1–2, 3, 18, 19
  reactive vs. proactive behaviors, 15–16
  self-assessment, of health condition, 3
Paxil, 10
peaches, 82

163

Made in the USA
Lexington, KY
14 May 2011